AFTER A
STROKE

A Support Book
for Patients, Caregivers,
Families and Friends

AFTER A
STROKE

A Support Book
for Patients, Caregivers,
Families and Friends

Geoffrey Donnan, M.D.
Carol Burton

NORTH ATLANTIC BOOKS
BERKELEY, CALIFORNIA

After a Stroke:
A Support Book for Patients, Caregivers, Families and Friends

Copyright © 1990 by Australian Brain Foundation. Copyright © 1992 "Feldenkrais Method" by Elizabeth Beringer and "A Naturopathic Perspective" by Marcus Laux. No portion of this book, except for brief review, may be reproduced in any form without written permission of the publisher. For information contact North Atlantic Books.

ISBN 1-55643-130-9

Published by
North Atlantic Books
P.O. Box 12327
Berkeley, CA 94712

First published in Australasia by Simon & Schuster Australia

Chapters 8 and 9 have been added in the American edition. They are not included in the index, and they do not represent the view of the Australian Brain Foundation.

Designed by Michelle Havenstein
Illustrated by Levent Efe
Typeset in Australia by Post Typesetters
Printed in the United States of America by Malloy Lithographing

After a Stroke: A Support Book for Patients, Caregivers, Families and Friends is sponsored by the Society for the Study of Native Arts and Sciences, a nonprofit educational corporation whose goals are to develop an educational and crosscultural perspective linking various scientific, social, and artistic fields; to nurture a holistic view of the arts, sciences, humanities, and healing; and to publish and distribute literature on the relationship of mind, body, and nature.

National Library of Australia Cataloguing in Publication Data

After a stroke : a support book for patients, caregivers, families and friends.

Includes index.
ISBN 1-55643-130-9

1. Cerebrovascular disease—Popular works.
I. Australian Brain Foundation.
616.81

Contents

Introduction

"I was two months pregnant. I hadn't been well for a while and was suffering from shocking headaches. Lights appeared in front of my eyes and I was getting a lot of cramps. The illness persisted and I was nervy and wanted something to calm me down, but the doctor advised against it because of possible danger to the baby.

One day, while I was reading, everything suddenly became blurry. I dropped the book I was holding. I couldn't talk. My hand went limp. I tried to get up and stumbled to the floor. The next thing I knew I was in hospital having tests. I was terrified of losing my baby. A CAT scan found a blood clot, but the doctors dared not operate. Instead I was given drugs to dissolve this unwanted intrusion."

Sue Latham used to be a heavy smoker consuming about two packets a day. The doctors now believe her stroke was a direct result of a combination of smoking and pregnancy, which causes the blood to thicken.

The memory of her stroke is still vivid in Sue's mind as she recalls what it was like afterwards to feel 'your brain scrambled, where you're trapped inside of yourself'.

Sue remained in a wheel chair for six months because her balance went completely. She had to learn to walk and talk all over again and it was three years before she could drive a car once more.

Therapies continue at home helping Sue to read and mix socially. It has been difficult to return to her love of essay writing and reading because her eyes still get blurry, particularly with small print. This is accentuated when she reads to her daughter, Emily, the 'miracle baby', who was eventually delivered by caesarean section and is now a healthy five-year-old. A weight increase is a result of depression, but Sue aims to fight that when the time is right.

Sue says that it has been and still is an immense ordeal and she feels vulnerable and in need of those who are closest to her. "I used to play on the stroke at first, but now I have greater independence. My mother and husband, Graham, have been strong thankfully and wonderfully supportive." Thanks also to the support of a carer, who herself had undergone the long haul back to 'normalcy', giving Sue the confidence that rehabilitation has worked for others. Sue continues to receive assistance through the Stroke Support Scheme which has been set up by the Australian Brain Foundation in Victoria.

When a person suffers a stroke, they need all the support and understanding they can get from those closest to them. Ignorance of stroke creates fear and misunderstanding which can build barriers between stroke persons and their supporters.

AFTER A STROKE has been written to inform and help anyone understand the many issues relating to stroke. As well as discussing exactly what a stroke is and how to prevent it, this book provides practical information on the important role of rehabilitation. The pathway to recovery from stroke is long and it is hoped that whether you are a person who has suffered a stroke, a carer, friend or health worker, or even consider yourself at risk, you will find this book to be a valuable resource.

Maxine Miller
Executive Director
Australian Brain Foundation

CHAPTER 1

What Is a Stroke?

Dr. Geoffrey A. Donnan

Stroke is the most common cause of death after heart disease and cancer in Western countries, yet most people do not understand the nature of stroke. When a person suffers a stroke, they need all the support and understanding they can get from those closest to them. Ignorance of stroke creates fear and misunderstanding which can build barriers between stroke persons and their supporters. By beginning this book with an outline of the structure of the brain and its blood supply, it is then easier to understand the causes of stroke and its effects on the body.

A stroke is caused by either blockage or rupture of a blood vessel within the brain or rupture of a blood vessel surrounding the brain. These events may then produce motor, sensory or intellectual dysfunction. This chapter describes the nature of a stroke, the effects are then described in subsequent chapters together with methods of rehabilitation.

THE STRUCTURE OF THE BRAIN

The brain is divided into three main components which are illustrated in Figure 1:

1. The *cerebrum* which is responsible for higher intellectual function, integration of sensory stimuli of all types, initiation of the final common pathway for movement and fine control of movement.

2. The *cerebellum* which is responsible for further control of movement and coordination.

3. The *brain stem* which is responsible for a variety of important functions including coordination of

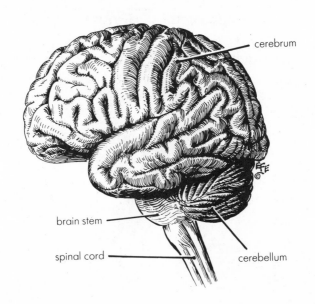

Figure 1 The three main regions of the brain

10

eye movements, and maintenance of balance, res-
piration and blood pressure.

THE BLOOD SUPPLY TO THE BRAIN

Blood circulation to the brain is via two major systems
as shown in Figure 2:

1. The largest amount of blood is conducted by the
   two *carotid arteries*, the pulsations of which may
   be readily felt in your own neck. These serve

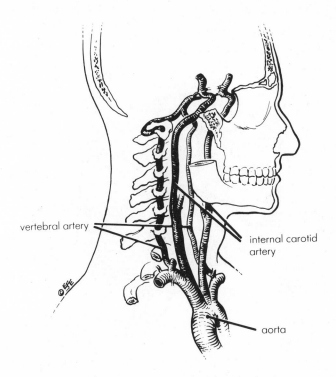

vertebral artery

internal carotid
artery

aorta

Figure 2 The major arteries leading to the brain

11

the front part of the brain, in fact, the major portion of both left and right hemispheres of the brain.

2. The two smaller *vertebral arteries* comprise the vertebrobasilar circulation system and serve the hind brain, reaching the brain by travelling in close association with the vertebral column at the back of the neck. These arteries serve the sensitive brain stem where centres for coordination of balance, eye movements, and swallowing are located. They also serve the cerebrum supplying blood to the hind portion of the brain which controls the integration of visual function. The mechanism by which these blood vessels may be affected by disease is outlined below.

WHAT CAUSES A STROKE?

Stroke may occur by one of three mechanisms:

1. Blockage of a blood vessel within the brain. Known as *cerebral infarction*, this may cause the death of the area of brain supplied by that particular blood vessel because of a lack of oxygen and other nutrients usually carried by the blood cells and plasma. (See Figure 3.)

2. Rupture of a blood vessel within the brain. Known as *cerebral haemorrhage*, this causes a distortion of the structure of the brain tissue because of pressure from the released blood. (See Figure 4.)

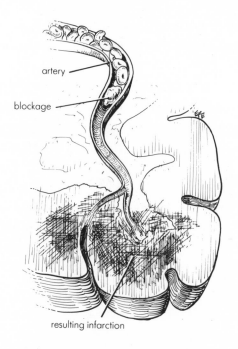

Figure 3 Cerebral infarction

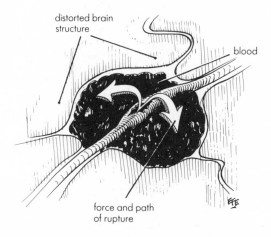

Figure 4 Cerebral haemorrhage

13

3. Rupture of a blood vessel into the space surrounding the brain, the *subarachnoid space*. It does not usually cause distortion of brain structure, but may cause spasm of the blood vessels nearby, thus impairing the blood supply to this area. This form of haemorrhage is called *subarachnoid haemorrhage*.

WHAT CAUSES BLOOD VESSELS TO BLOCK OR RUPTURE?

Blood vessels in the brain most commonly block because a blood clot has broken off and travelled along an artery up into the brain until the vessel size allows no further passage. The source of the clot is usually as follows:

1. The *internal carotid artery* where deposits of fatty material (*atheroma*) cause narrowing of the artery (*stenosis*). The site of this narrowing is most often at the point where the common carotid artery divides into its internal and external branches. (See Figure 5.) This artery can be felt in the neck at about the angle of the jaw. The narrowing of the artery at this point disturbs the pattern of blood flow and creates turbulence. This makes the formation of clots more likely and, if they do occur, they may break off and be swept along the artery into the brain. Sometimes the degree of arterial narrowing at this point may become critical and complete occlusion or closure occurs. If the circulation is unable to be re-established

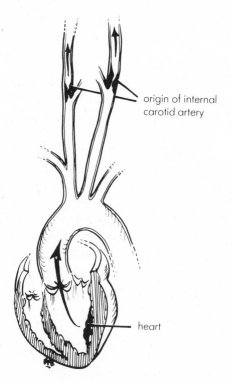

origin of internal
carotid artery

heart

Figure 5 Two common sites of origin of clot formation

via other blood vessels (if one vessel blocks, another can often provide a detour), then cerebral infarction in the region of the internal carotid artery will occur.

2. The *heart*. For this to occur, the heart usually has a major functional or structural abnormality, such as an abnormal rhythm (*atrial fibrillation*), recent heart attack (*myocardial infarction*) or a generalised weakness of heart muscle (*cardio-myopathy*). Clots form in much the same way as within the carotid artery due to turbulence of

15

blood flow or alteration of the characteristics of the surface against which the blood is flowing. (See also Figure 5.)

Rupture of blood vessels is less common and is usually due to a defect in the vessel wall. This may occur in three major ways (see Figure 6):

1. The effects of high blood pressure (*hypertension*) over a prolonged period of time cause damage to small blood vessels deep within the brain. These vessels are fragile and develop regions of damage known as *lipohyalinosis*. In many instances these vessels may block to produce small areas of infarction (known as lacunes because of their small, lake-like appearance) or, on other occasions, they

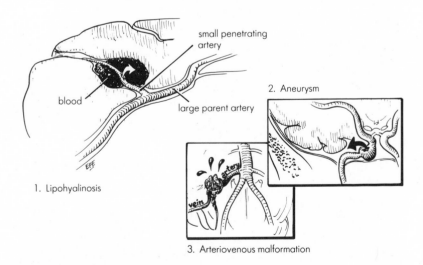

Figure 6 Three major causes of cerebral haemorrhage

may rupture thus producing a cerebral haemorrhage.

2. Rupture of a defect in the wall of vessels surrounding the brain. The defect is in the form of an outpouching of the artery and is called an *aneurysm*, or *Berry aneurysm*. The vessels lie in the subarachnoid space and hence the haemorrhage is termed *subarachnoid haemorrhage*.

3. Rupture of malformed blood vessels within the brain. These malformations occur at the junction of the arterial and venous systems and are hence termed *arteriovenous malformations*, or *A–V malformations*.

WHAT FACTORS PREDISPOSE ONE TO DEVELOP A STROKE?

There are a well-recognised series of factors which may predispose an individual to develop a stroke. These are as follows:

- Increase in age

- High blood pressure (hypertension)

- Smoking

- Diabetes

- Other factors such as high cholesterol, obesity, lack of exercise, and stress. These have not been as clearly established as the first four factors.

Preventative measures may be taken to minimise these risks. This most important topic will be addressed in more detail in later chapters.

SYMPTOMS OF SMALL WARNING STROKES

Approximately 50 per cent of patients who subsequently have a stroke due to blockage of a blood vessel (*cerebral infarction*) have a small warning episode termed a *transient ischaemic attack* or TIA. This may often be of the same clinical pattern as the eventual stroke but of briefer duration. Many of these warnings last for minutes only, although occasionally they may last for several hours, or even up to 24 hours. TIAs may be located in either the carotid or vertebrobasilar circulation systems. The symptoms which may be experienced are as follows:

In the region of the carotid arteries

Fleeting blindness or blurring of vision in one eye

Some refer to this as *transient monocular blindness* (TMB) to more specifically restrict the symptom to one eye only. Another commonly used medical term is *amaurosis fugax*. Typically there may be a sudden complete loss of vision in one eye lasting for a few seconds or minutes only, or the onset may be like a curtain "descending or ascending" from above or below. Very occasionally it may cross from one side to the other although this is less common. It is often helpful for diagnosis if the person covers one eye or the other at the time of the incident to be certain that one eye only is involved. Such certainty of location places the episode of ischaemia in the carotid rather than the vertebrobasilar circulation system since a branch of the carotid artery (opthalmic) supplies the eye, and is therefore in effect "a window" to the carotid circulation system. Amaurosis fugax should not be confused with episodes of homonymous heminiopia described later.

Speech disturbance

When an episode of circulatory impairment affects the left hemisphere of the brain where the speech centre is located, speech disturbances of various types may result (*aphasias*). When the front portion of the brain is affected, expression of speech may be impaired (*expressive aphasia*). Typically a sufferer complains: "I knew what I wanted to say but was unable to say it." Sometimes words of a similar type but different meaning may be produced. For example: "I wicked up my pat", really meaning "I picked up my hat". When the hind portion of the brain is affected, comprehension or understanding may be impaired (*receptive aphasia*). During these periods free flow of speech may occur but it may be quite nonsensical (*jargon aphasia*). Mixtures of these speech disturbances may also occur.

Weakness or paralysis of face, arm or leg

The most common form of TIA in the carotid circulation system involves a brief episode of weakness or clumsiness affecting face, arm or leg separately or in combination. Typically the case description may be of an episode of weakness affecting the person's right arm and leg together with speech disturbance, resulting in an object being dropped, the limb feeling heavy or even numb or tingling. Occasionally the weakness may be so profound that the limbs on one side of the body are unable to be moved at all for brief periods and need to be lifted by the good arm. At times these symptoms may occur on repeated occasions. On other occasions the symptoms might be so minimal that a brief period of clumsiness only is experienced, for example, while using a knife or fork or writing.

In the region of the vertebral arteries

Here the symptoms may be more variable since sensitive areas of brain function in the brain stem may be affected. Specifically, balance together with speech and vision may often be affected.

Vertigo

This denotes a spinning sensation and is usually experienced in conjunction with other symptoms described below. Vertigo in the absence of other symptoms is more often due to an inner ear disturbance than TIA. Typically with TIAs, vertigo is present continuously regardless of head position whereas vertigo associated with inner ear disturbance is very much positionally related.

Double vision

Objects may suddenly appear to be double in a horizontal or vertical sense. It may be more marked when looking in one direction as opposed to another.

Facial numbness or weakness

This usually occurs in conjunction with speech disturbance described below.

Slurring of speech

In contrast to carotid circulation system speech disturbance, disturbance due to vertebrobasilar or hindbrain ischaemia results in a slurring of speech, often with an accompanying sensation that the tongue is moving clumsily. Alternatively the tongue is described as "thick".

Swallowing difficulty

Occasionally this may accompany the speech disturbance described above.

Arm or leg weakness or paralysis

This may occur in a similar way as that associated with the carotid circulation. However, the symptoms may occasionally involve one side followed by the other side of the body in quick succession and if this is so, then it clearly separates the symptoms from carotid circulation system problems.

Loss of balance

This may occur as a separate entity to the vertigo described above and may manifest itself in a tendency to veer to one side or the other, or in a generalised difficulty in remaining upright.

Nausea and vomiting

When this occurs it is more often in conjunction with vertigo as described above.

Other visual disturbances

Apart from double vision, difficulty may be experienced seeing one or other of the visual fields to the left or right. The sudden onset of this difficulty may result in the patient being able to see only half of the dual field before them no matter where they look. This should be carefully distinguished from monocular amarosis fugax, described under carotid circulation system TIAs, and may be distinguished by covering each eye separately. In the case of impairment of half of the visual field (*homonymous heminiopia*), this symptom will be present on covering either eye. In case of monocular amarosis fugax, covering the unaffected eye will result in an inability to see anything while covering the affected eye will result in normal vision being experienced in the opposite unaffected eye.

SYMPTOMS OF ESTABLISHED STROKES

The symptoms of established strokes may be subdivided into three main forms of stroke.

1. Cerebral infarction

2. Cerebral haemorrhage

3. Subarachnoid haemorrhage.

Cerebral infarction

Symptoms of cerebral infarction (due to blockage of a blood vessel) are as for small warning strokes described above except that the changes are permanent.

Cerebral haemorrhage

Episodes of cerebral haemorrhage (due to rupture of a blood vessel within the brain) are usually not preceded by small warning episodes as for cerebral infarction. It is usually a once only development of weakness affecting one side of the body including speech if the left side of the brain is involved. A depression in consciousness is a frequent accompaniment. The damage caused is usually greater than that of cerebral infarction and the mortality rate is higher.

Subarachnoid haemorrhage

Due to rupture of a blood vessel in the space surrounding the brain, this haemorrhage is sometimes preceded by a small "warning leak" where the sudden onset of an extremely severe headache together with neck stiffness may be experienced. Irritation from light (*photophobia*) may also be a problem. The beginning of the subarachnoid haemorrhage itself is associated with the usually sudden commencement of the worst headache ever experienced by that person, often combined with reduced consciousness and neck stiffness.

HOW IS A STROKE DIAGNOSED?

Stroke diagnosis may be divided into five major sections:

1. Clinical assessment

2. CAT scan

3. Duplex ultrasound

4. Angiography

5. Other investigations.

Clinical assessment

This is the first and most important part of the diagnostic process. Your doctor will be able to assess which part of the brain has been affected by taking details of how the stroke developed and performing a careful clinical examination. The stroke type can then be loosely categorised into either cerebral infarction, haemorrhage or subarachnoid haemorrhage. Alternatively, if a transient ischaemic attack (TIA) has occurred, the arterial region affected may be identified by a careful description of the symptoms involved. Your doctor will then be able to arrange appropriate investigations.

CAT scan (Computerised Axial Tomography)

This is the next step to be performed to confirm the site of the stroke and to definitively diagnose whether it was a cerebral infarction (see Figure 7) or haemorrhage (see Figure 8). In general when the CAT scan is performed within 24 hours following the event, little change is seen on the CAT scan when cerebral infarction has occurred. However, in the case of cerebral haemorrhage the change is seen immediately. Similarly with subarachnoid haemorrhage blood may be seen in the subarachnoid space. The blood is shown as an intense white area on the CAT scan which is extremely easy to see.

The CAT scan itself is a computerised form of multiple X-rays performed in a radial fashion around the head. Its introduction in the late 1970s has revolutionised stroke diagnosis together with many other neurological conditions.

Duplex ultrasound of carotid arteries

Since one of the major causes of cerebral infarction is a clot arising from the carotid artery in the neck, duplex ultrasound study of this region may reveal an area of narrowing (stenosis) of the artery itself. This technology involves the transmission and reception of

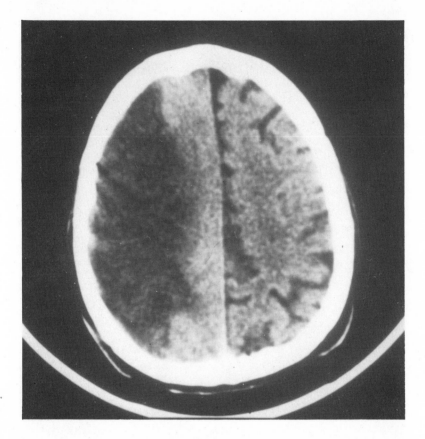

Figure 7 CAT scan of a cerebral infarction

ultrasound signals to the arterial system via a transducer placed over the skin surface near the carotid artery. (See Figure 9.) It may be combined with a spectral analysis of the flow characteristics of blood passing through an area of narrowing. The reliability of this technology is now great enough to use it as a major screening method to establish the status of the carotid arterial system in the neck in patients who have had brief warning strokes.

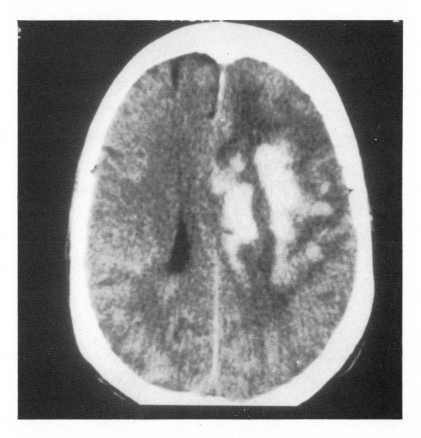

Figure 8 CAT scan of a cerebral haemorrhage

Angiography

The principle of this technique is to introduce into the arterial system a small catheter through which may be injected a radio-opaque dye. This is usually done by a small skin puncture in the groin after a local anaesthetic has been injected into the same region. An X-ray will then outline the inner structure of the artery so that any defects may be identified. In recent years

27

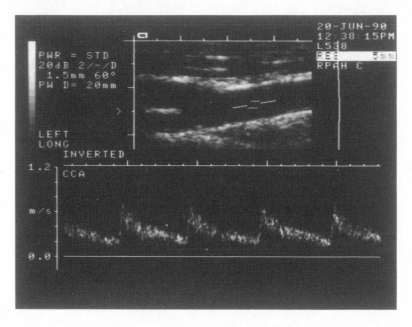

Figure 9 Duplex ultrasound of the carotid artery

this procedure has undergone such significant techno-
logical advances that only small amounts of dye need
to be injected because the resulting X-ray image is
enhanced by computerised techniques. This is termed
digital subtraction angiography (DSA). By using this technique, the carotid and vertebrobasilar arteries in the
neck as well as the blood vessels within the brain itself
may be clearly seen. (See Figure 10.) It is most often
used after a TIA or minor stroke so that the mechanism

28

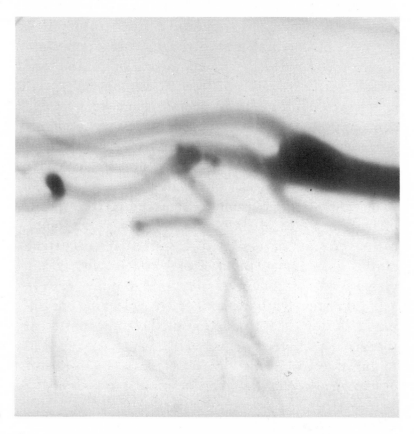

Figure 10 A carotid angiogram

by which the event occurred can be established. For example, the angiogram may reveal an almost complete blockage of the internal carotid artery in the neck responsible for the generation of clots which have broken off and subsequently lodged in a blood vessel within the brain to produce the symptoms described. Once the mechanism of the stroke has been established, appropriate management of the condition can be planned. This may include the use of anticoagulants

29

(blood thinning agents) or surgery (see treatment). In the case of cerebral haemorrhage, angiography may also be used to identify any malformations of the blood vessels (arteriovenous malformations or AVMs). In people with subarachnoid haemorrhage in whom the damage is modest, angiography is necessary to identify the area of arterial defect (aneurysm) since in many instances this may be clipped by a neurosurgeon to prevent further episodes of bleeding.

In general, angiography is reserved for the specific indications outlined above since it may cause complications in some instances, such as the rare occurrence of the development of a stroke in its own right by virtue of the introduction of a foreign object into the arterial system (catheter and/or dye); bleeding or bruising at the site of introduction of the catheter (usually the groin); or very occasionally an allergic reaction to the dye itself. For this latter reason, any history of known allergies should be mentioned to your doctor.

Other investigations

If the heart is suspected as the source of the clot, then investigations of the heart may be appropriate. These include a standard *electrocardiograph* (ECG) to determine if the rhythm is regular and whether any underlying heart attack has occurred. An ultrasound of the heart (*echocardiograph*) may also be undertaken in a way similar to the carotid artery investigation. This may detect areas of abnormal heart movement or the presence of a clot. A *chest x-ray* may be useful to look at the outline of the heart. Another routine investigation is a *blood count* to detect any anaemia, abnormal blood thickening or arterial infections (arteritis).

MORE DETAIL ABOUT STROKE TYPES

Further information about stroke types may help you understand some of the events experienced by a stroke person. The type of stroke which has developed will very much influence what tests are done, what sort of treatment is given and what sort of problems may be experienced during the recovery period and rehabilitation. First, let's consider the commonest form of stroke, cerebral infarction which, as outlined previously, is due to blockage of blood vessels within the brain.

Cerebral infarction

Occlusion or closure may affect both major and minor (penetrating) blood vessels. The location of these blood vessels and the effects of occlusion may be seen in Figure 11.

Major blood vessel occlusion

The most common blood vessel involved is the middle cerebral artery which supplies blood to much of the cerebral hemisphere. In the left hemisphere, occlusion or closure of this blood vessel or one of its branches will result in a combination of speech disturbance (*aphasia* — see previous discussion) and weakness affecting the right side of the body, involving face, arm and leg. If the occlusion is located to the rear of the left hemisphere, difficulty with comprehension will result. Occlusions located near the front result in difficulty in speech expression. In the right hemisphere, occlusion of the middle cerebral artery or its branches may result in a marked neglect of the left side of the body together with a weakness affecting face, arm or leg. If the weakness is quite mild there may be difficulty with dressing (*dressing dyspraxia*) together with other difficulties in appreciating three-dimensional concepts. Occlusion of the front cerebral artery, producing infarction of the frontal lobe may result in a profound lethargy and lack of desire to initiate any rehabilitation.

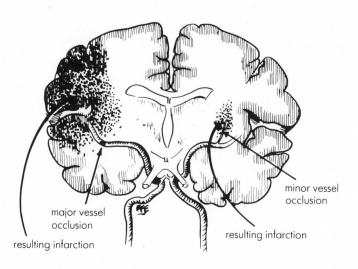

Figure 11 Major and minor penetrating vessel occlusion resulting in areas of infarction

Occlusion of the rear cerebral arteries produces a variety of problems involving visual disturbance. Specifically *homonymous heminiopia* (inability to see out of one side of one's visual field) may be common.

Small blood vessel (penetrator) occlusion

Since small, penetrating blood vessels radiate up into the brain from its base, they do not usually reach the outer surface (cortex of the brain). Since the cortex contains most of the integrative functions of the brain concerned with speech, awareness, sensation and/or visual integration, occlusion or closure of these small vessels usually results in involvement of motor (movement) and sensory tracts only as they course through the deep parts of the brain. Therefore, unlike occlusions of the major blood vessels, such signs as speech disturbance, loss of awareness, and visual disturbance are rarely present. This makes rehabilitation a much simpler task.

Involvement of a single penetrating blood vessel produces a small area of infarction only. (See Figure 11.) This area has been termed *lacune* from its lakelike appearance in pathological specimens. The features of strokes due to a single, small, blood vessel occlusion such as these are therefore called *lacunar syndromes*. The most common of these is *pure motor hemiplegia* which involves weakness of face, arm and leg equally without any sensory involvement nor any impairment in speech or other cognitive functions. The outlook for rehabilitation in these cases is therefore better than most other forms of stroke.

Brain stem damage

Brain stem infarcts (areas of damage) produce more permanent disabilities similar to the signs and symptoms produced during vertebrobasilar TIAs but are longer lasting (see previous discussion). One of the major characteristics of brain stem infarction or lesions of the brain stem is the crossed nature of the signs produced. Due to the nature of the arterial pathways concerned with the brain stem, the weakness may affect one side of the face together with the opposite side of the body. Similarly, sensory loss may follow the same pattern. Another feature of brain stem involvement may be double vision, vertigo, nausea, vomiting, slurring of speech and swallowing difficulty. Since the vertebral arteries join eventually to the rear cerebral arteries, homonymous heminiopia, or inability to see out of one side of one's visual field, may also be a feature.

If the cerebellum is involved, marked loss of balance (*ataxia*) may occur. Occasionally the cerebellum only is involved so this may be the only symptom produced.

Cerebral haemorrhage

Similar symptoms to an infarction or blockage may be produced by the presence of cerebral haemorrhage in either left or right hemisphere or brain stem. Often the haemorrhage tends to have a more devastating effect than infarction with resultant depression in consciousness although with small haemorrhages excellent recovery is common. Hence, left hemisphere haemorrhages produce speech disturbances with weakness affecting the right side, right hemisphere haemorrhages produce neglect or loss of awareness of the left side together with weakness involving face, arm and leg, and difficulties with appreciating three-dimensional concepts and dressing. Brain stem haemorrhages may also produce the same array of symptoms as a cerebral infarction.

Subarachnoid haemorrhage

The array of problems produced by a subarachnoid haemorrhage depends upon the actual position of haemorrhage. As for infarction and intracerebral haemorrhage, each hemisphere and vascular region may be affected by a blood vessel spasm secondary to the haemorrhage, producing the same array of clinical problems as an infarction or cerebral haemorrhage. If the subarachnoid haemorrhage is confined entirely to the space surrounding the brain without the complication of a blood vessel spasm within the brain itself, no specific neurological signs will be produced except that of neck stiffness and perhaps some reduction of consciousness.

GENERAL COMMENTS ON THE DEVELOPMENT OF A STROKE

While the onset of most forms of stroke is quite sudden, occasionally a gradual progression over a period of minutes may be experienced. Once the stroke has reached its nadir and the damage has been done, a period of spontaneous resolution of the signs produced tends to occur. This is because the area of damage eventually is somewhat smaller than the original insult and also, other parts of the brain take over the work of that area damaged. This is a slow process and is very much aided by rehabilitation. This will be covered in subsequent sections in this book.

CHAPTER 2

Consequences of a Stroke

Dr. Michael M. Saling

PSYCHOLOGICAL FUNCTION AFTER A STROKE

When a stroke produces permanent change to brain areas which are involved in the regulation of psychological processes such as the production and understanding of language, reasoning, planning, judging, or emotion, the stroke-affected person engages in a massive and valiant struggle to compensate for the void left by a loss of function. This struggle may itself produce emotional upheaval, or strange behaviour, which may be incomprehensible to others. We refer to these compensatory attempts as the "catastrophic reaction" — literally an attempt to cope with a catastrophic loss of function, the suddenness of which is unparalleled in other illnesses affecting the brain.

The catastrophic reaction is an extremely variable phenomenon. It may be quite obvious, manifesting itself as explosive anger, frustration, or uncharacteristic annoyance, particularly in those who have lost the capacity to express themselves by means of speech. Alternatively, the stroke person may become depressed or withdrawn. The way in which the reaction is expressed is intimately dependent on the person's personality, and it may even be modified by the location of the stroke itself.

Another major factor which determines behaviour after a stroke is the type of psychological loss that was suffered. The loss is often referred to as a "deficit". Accordingly, the psychological condition after stroke is often described as if something has been subtracted — without language, without recognition, without memory. To a certain extent this way of viewing psychological function after a stroke is correct. However, it fails to capture the idea that there is some reorganisation of the functions that remain. This reorganisation is not chaotic, but seeks to maximise adaptation to a changed world. The great neuropsychologist, Alexandr Luria, identified this tendency as a fundamental property of the brain, the struggle of an altered system to reach a "constant end" (the fulfilment of strivings, the realisation of intentions which are essential in the process of adaptation) by "variable means" (compensation, reorganisation of preserved function).

We know very little about the ways in which psychological systems reorganise themselves after events such as strokes. It is probably the case that the nature of the loss suffered plays an important role in determining the nature of these attempts. One of the best ways of conveying these ideas to the reader is to consider some actual examples, concentrating on the kinds of loss that are most frequently studied by clinical neuropsychologists, namely, cognitive loss.

LANGUAGE LOSS AFTER A LEFT HEMISPHERE STROKE

Although the two hemispheres of the brain appear to be physical mirror images of one another (ignoring, for the moment, some minor structural differences that have been found), they are quite different when viewed through neuropsychological eyes. The so-called "dominant" hemisphere (the left hemisphere in most people) is primarily concerned with language function. It is better than the right hemisphere at expressing itself in terms of language (speaking and writing), at understanding the spoken and written word, and at remembering information which is presented in a verbal form. When the left hemisphere is involved in a stroke, the most frequent consequence is a loss in some aspect of language function.

A case history

N.Y. was a healthy and active tennis coach when he suffered a sudden occlusion (blockage) in the left internal carotid artery. The internal carotid artery is the main supply route to the middle cerebral artery, which in turn supplies blood to a very large part of the lateral surface of the left hemisphere.

Shortly after this event, *N.Y.* could utter only one or two words. He could not even repeat words or simple phrases that were spoken to him (that is, he could not imitate simple speech). Further, *N.Y.* could not carry out simple actions that were requested of him, despite the fact that his capacity to carry out the relevant movements was not impaired. In short, *N.Y.* could neither use, nor comprehend language at a basic level. This condition is the most severe form of language loss seen after a stroke, and is referred to as *global aphasia* (without language).

As the days went by, there was a rapid recovery of *N.Y.*'s language function. His speech regained its fluency, and he once again began to use complete, well-constructed sentences instead of the isolated words that he had been restricted to after his stroke. However, he would frequently make mistakes in the "pronunciation" of words. These mistakes suggested he was having some trouble with the construction of words he wanted to say. More specifically, he sometimes chose sound patterns that were inappropriate, and words would pop out in an incorrect form: instead of the word "dish", for example, he might say "beshess". "Beshess" is an approximation to the actual word, that is, a paraphasia, literally meaning to speak alongside.

Sometimes, *N.Y.* would be completely unable to find a word that he needed, and prominent pauses would appear in his spontaneous speech. When this occurred, he would often try to "speak around" the word he could not find, and his spoken language came to sound rather vague and empty.

As *N.Y.* recovered further, it became clear that he had lost the ability to do fairly simple arithmetic calculations. Also, he could no longer tell the difference between left and right. However, the loss that troubled him most was the inability to read and write. In other words, as a result of his stroke, he had acquired *alexia* (without reading) and *agraphia* (without writing).

Up to this point, the post-stroke history of *N.Y.* is quite typical of individuals who suffer strokes in a particular branch of the middle cerebral artery known as the inferior division. Alexia with agraphia is a serious outcome, and is usually permanent. However, the story of *N.Y.* takes an unexpected turn.

When *N.Y.*'s reading difficulty was subjected to detailed neuropsychological study, it was found that he could read certain words. These words have in common the fact that their spelling corresponds closely with their sound structure; one can read them accurately by simply sounding out the individual letters, in much the same way that a young child or a very unskilled reader might do. And this was the strategy that *N.Y.* used. If he was presented with an irregular word (where there is no direct correspondence between spelling and sound structure, as is the case with words such as argue, debt, gauge) his reading ability completely disappeared.

This letter-by-letter reading process is not characteristic of the syndrome of alexia with agraphia. The process itself suggests that the patient cannot recognise words on the basis of their visual appearance, but rather, recognition takes place on the basis of the sound of the word. In rather more technical terms, one could say that letter-by-letter readers cannot access their internal word stores by visual means, but they can do so by auditory means.

Now we know that reading in terms of the sound structure of words is the more basic process of the two; visual access reading occurs later in the development of reading skills. This has implications for the reorganisation and recovery of reading after a stroke. Unlike most people who suffer from alexia with agraphia, *N.Y.* eventually recovered a great deal of his reading ability, probably because he was able to make use of his preserved ability to recognise words by auditory means.

A brain scan showed that the stroke had occurred in the territory between the middle cerebral artery and a neighbouring artery known as the posterior cerebral artery.

Important issues

There are a number of issues emerging from the case of *N.Y.*

1. Although the neuropsychological loss may appear to be very severe in the early days after a stroke, a degree of recovery may occur. This is not invariable, but the possibility should be borne in mind.

2. In some cases, there may be unsuspected preservation of function which could serve as a basis

for some degree of functional reorganisation and recovery. This may become evident after careful neuropsychological examination in the late stages of recovery.

NEGLECT AFTER A RIGHT HEMISPHERE STROKE

The neuropsychological disorders that occur after left hemisphere strokes are usually highly specific and easily described. Similarly, the patient's emotional state after a left hemisphere stroke can be readily interpreted in terms of the concept of the catastrophic reaction. However, in the case of right hemisphere strokes, the resulting neuropsychological change is more difficult to understand. Emotional states emerge which are bewildering because they appear to signal a fundamental change in personality; they are completely uncharacteristic, and may even seem a little bizarre.

The right hemisphere of the brain has some rather basic language functions, but it is fundamentally concerned with matters non-verbal. These appear to include the understanding of music and other meaningful but non-linguistic sounds (for example, the rush of water, a dog's bark, and the like). Foremost among the documented functions of the right hemisphere is its role in the understanding of space.

The idea of space plays a major role in our daily lives. It is the basis of the way in which we find routes, appreciate the position of our bodies in relation to other objects around us, understand and execute drawings, construct houses, and remember faces. When a stroke affects the right hemisphere of the brain, various forms of spatial deficit may occur. One of the most fundamental expressions of a spatial deficit is the phenomenon of neglect.

Neglect is not a single loss, but rather, a constellation of losses, which are characterised by the fact that the stroke-affected person does not take note of, or perform actions within, the space to the left of the body midline. A variety of emotional changes may also be associated with neglect. The following is a list of behavioural changes that may signal the presence of neglect.

- Dressing only the right side of the body
- Reading from the middle of a printed page towards the right
- Continually bumping the left side of the body against doorposts
- Eating only off the right side of the plate
- Failing to utilise the left arm for bimanual activities.

This list could be expanded endlessly. The essential feature is that the left side of space, including the left side of the stroke person's own body, is ignored. This occurs despite the fact that the person is able to receive sensory input from the left side of space, and there is no abnormality of movement on the left.

Some stroke persons develop strange feelings about the left arm, and may even deny ownership of the arm. The feeling that the left arm belongs to someone else can be quite overpowering, and will be maintained despite the most obvious evidence to the contrary. The impression that the left arm is a foreign object may be so strong that the patient attempts to throw the arm away, claiming that it is merely pinned to his body. Reactions such as these appear to be quite irrational, and may even be mistaken for psychiatric problems. It is perhaps fortunate that they seldom persist into the chronic phase of recovery. Sometimes denial may become a more general feature of the condition, and the patient may quite emphatically deny any illness or disability. These reactions can be usefully understood as extremely primitive forms of the catastrophic reaction. Apathy rather than a sense of frustration may be the persisting emotional state.

SOME PERSPECTIVE

Not all stroke persons suffer neuropsychological changes, and some have barely noticeable changes. The degree of change depends on a large number of factors which include the size and position of the stroke, the age of the person, and the presence of left-handedness in the family (where there is a family history of left-handedness, neuropsychological recovery may be more rapid and complete).

CHAPTER 3

Stroke: Its Effect on the Family

Carol Burton

Strokes are suffered by individuals, yet consequences of stroke are far reaching, causing great distress to immediate family members or partners who have to shoulder the emotional and practical burdens, the interruptions to family life and role changes. A stroke has wide ramifications touching every aspect of life: it affects intimate relationships, friendships, social networks, recreational and vocational activities. It may force adaptation to a completely new way of life and new kinds of relationships. The effects of a stroke are complex and few "outsiders" can appreciate the effort involved in regaining independence or the strain on the family during the period of the illness.

Since the severity of a stroke may range from mild to profound, the effects of a stroke may vary from subtle behavioural alterations to significant intellectual, memory and behavioural changes. Whatever the extent of these changes, they are likely to contribute to a lessening of the quality of life. Adjustments to the effects of the stroke and the threats to one's sense of identity and self-worth will have to be made. There may be a period of mourning and trying to learn to live with losses: loss of control of body functions, and physical and motor weakness; loss of independence; changes in self-concept; loss in self-esteem. The person may fear total loss of control; loss of family support for fear that they may regard him or her as inadequate, or a useless burden; and may also fear the possibility of death. The level of awareness of deficits determines the emotional reactions. Initially, most experience a period of increased emotionality. Certain strokes may also result in increased tearfulness which is not associated with feelings of sadness and is a cause of embarrassment.

Generally, the more severe the damage resulting from stroke, the less awareness or insight that will be shown. Some people who have suffered a stroke may be aware that they are less efficient and more dependent than before the stroke but have lost the capacity to appreciate why this is so. They are often unaware of their deficiencies. With mild strokes minimal emotional and personality alterations are experienced but there may be sensitivity to reduced mental efficiency, diminished control of emotions, clumsiness, slowness, expressive difficulties and fatigue and this can lead to increased anxiety and depression.

Some of the behavioural and emotional reactions

are directly due to brain dysfunction caused by the stroke (such as pathological crying) and others are due to the person's reactions to the perceived changes, but generally there is a complex interaction between the psychological changes that occur as a direct result of the brain not functioning properly and those psychological reactions that reflect how the person views these changes and their ramifications. Before describing the behavioural problems that are most likely to contribute to family problems, it may be helpful to review common reactions of family members to stroke.

COMMON REACTIONS OF FAMILY MEMBERS

The acute stage

Initially the family goes through a period of acute shock and disbelief at what has happened. The event may seem unreal, feelings may be numbed. There is anxiety about the possibility of death, and commonly, the first reaction on arriving at hospital is one of relief that the person has not died. The major hope is that the person will recover irrespective of any long-term consequences.

Although relieved that the person has not died, there may be a lingering fear of the possibility of death. Such fears must be faced at a time of increased sensitivity. Some relatives may find themselves thinking that it may be better for the person to die in order to avoid the frustrations and difficulties that lie ahead but often these thoughts are suppressed because of the feelings of guilt they arouse.

Apart from anxiety about death, and worries about the future, relatives have to endure watching the suffering of someone they love and many stand by in helpless frustration, afraid and ignorant of what has been happening. Communication difficulties with medical staff may add to their distress.

The confusion and disorientation stroke persons show can be quite stressful. Sometimes the person may be verbally abusive or physically aggressive and relatives have a difficult time deciding whether this is a true reflection of feelings or not. This behaviour, so out of character, may be quite frightening. Another source of stress is the child-like behaviour that may be observed. People who have been self-sufficient in their daily lives before the stroke become complaining, demanding and dependent during hospitalisation. Unaccustomed to such behaviour, the family becomes alternatively confused or angry. They want to respond to the person's needs but are bewildered by the uncharacteristic demands. Relatives become angry when the person does not give them credit for their efforts and continues to behave childishly. Such behaviour is not deliberate.

Family members may feel guilty about the occurrence of the stroke, wondering whether there was anything they might have done to prevent it, or they may feel guilty for feeling helpless, or not reacting as they would have liked. At some stage, relatives feel guilty about the anger and resentment that inevitably surfaces. The anger derives from feelings of injustice ("why me?"), and anger may arise from resentment of the person who has had the stroke for causing such emotional pain, worry and disruption. Sometimes, too, those with religious beliefs are angry that God has allowed such a terrible thing to happen.

Such reactions are normal and in spite of the high degree of stress, most people find the inner resources needed to cope with the pressures and demands of the situation. Family members' emotional reactions will vary widely and fluctuate frequently. There will be good days and bad, times when progress exceeds expectations and times when nothing appears to have happened. Emotions may range from shock and disbelief to denial of reality (denying the stroke has happened, fantasising that the person will return to their former self). There may be anger, guilt, feelings of sadness, loss and grief. All or any of these feelings may be experienced and they may last for a short time or may last for considerably longer before the grief resolves. At the same time the adjustments to, and restructuring of, life commences. The whole process is analogous to, but more complicated than, the grieving that follows bereavement.

Rehabilitation stage

Some people are only temporarily disabled by stroke and are soon discharged from the acute hospital. Others are transferred to a rehabilitation hospital or centre which they attend as inpatients or day patients. It is at this stage that the residual effects of the stroke (particularly the behavioural) become most apparent.

Active rehabilitation produces renewed hope that recovery will be full and the person will return to their former self. This may be true for some, but for most, recovery is a long, slow, frustrating process. Sometimes relatives feel progress might be more rapid if the person tried harder (generally, the person is doing the best he/she can given their disabilities) or could be more independent if only the relative knew how to help. Certainly, the active involvement of relatives is crucial for the well-being, support and encouragement of the person, and their understanding will promote a constructive adjustment to the illness and will make reintegration into the family and community easier. Such involvement and understanding may help to establish more realistic short and long-term goals.

BEHAVIOURAL CHANGES AFFECTING FAMILY INTEGRITY

Every individual is different and affected differently by stroke but among the most common and troublesome effects of stroke are the personality changes. These frequently overshadow the intellectual changes. The behavioural alterations vary in degree, sometimes appearing as little more than a slight coarsening of behaviour and sometimes appearing as gross changes with limited behavioural or impulse control. Pre-existing personality characteristics may be enhanced.

Typically, the person with marked personality change displays a child-like egocentricity (as if the world revolves around them) which is associated with diminished self-awareness, social insensitivity, tactlessness, and an inability to consider the feelings of others. If a person cannot appreciate the social niceties, he or she is likely to behave in ways that are likely to embarrass relatives or friends. If he or she cannot understand socially meaningful gestures, facial expressions and the reactions of others, he or she may not appreciate when their partner is tired or unhappy, or be aware that their behaviour is inappropriate. Spouses find the lack of consideration and inability to provide emotional support very draining. It becomes too much of an effort or embarrassing to attend social outings or family gatherings and gradually the family become increasingly isolated as old friends and even other relatives stop visiting. The spouse may feel exhausted and unappreciated.

Impaired ability to control behaviour may also be very trying. Increased impulsivity is one aspect of decreased control and affects all areas of life from handling money (impulsive and frequently unnecessary purchases) to overeating (so that the spouse has to resort to hiding food). There may be sexual impulsivity with inappropriate sexual advances to visitors or strangers. Stopping any behaviour (for example, laughter at a joke) may be difficult, just as initiating activities may be impossible without prompting.

Physical restlessness and agitation are also problems associated with diminished control. It may become irritating to family members when the person doesn't stop fidgeting or pacing and the restlessness of some may result in wandering out and getting lost, so that the family has to be ever vigilant.

Temper outbursts and abusive language triggered for no apparent reason are hard to handle. Impatience increases irritability and the likelihood of temper outbursts.

There may be an inability to adjust to anything new or out of the ordinary and small changes may make a person anxious, irritable and depressed. Consequently, new experiences are avoided and there is a tendency to stick to an unvarying routine. This inability to act spontaneously and flexibly can be a problem when having to confront new tasks or social demands. Where problems with planning and organisation exist, there is a need for external guidance and support and here a routine is beneficial. While some people are able to accomplish familiar routines with little or no help and only need assistance when undertaking new or complex tasks, others may require constant reminding to accomplish simple activities of daily living such as changing their clothes or brushing their teeth. It is not wilful laziness or a lack of motivation and under such circumstances, family members should not feel guilty about providing the structure and support that is needed.

What may puzzle the family more, is the person's apparent inability to learn from mistakes even when the same errors lead repeatedly to trouble. Under normal circumstances, people are allowed to make mistakes because they learn valuable lessons from them. With the person who has suffered a stroke, the family may have to step in where appropriate to protect the person from potential danger.

Other neurologically based emotional changes that

families find difficult to tolerate are apathy (an inability to initiate activity), silly childish behaviour, and denial of limitations. The misbehaviour is not deliberate or meant to annoy (although it undeniably does so) although it may be used to ensure attention.

Most moderate to severely impaired stroke survivors are dependent on their families for some physical care or financial support. Strong emotional dependency ties may develop as a result of feelings of inadequacy insecurity, fear of deterioration or abandonment. Many attempt to maintain a sense of control or authority by forcing their spouses to wait on them but this is likely to backfire and result in greater invalidism and dependency. Some, more mobile than others, fear abandonment and follow their spouses wherever they go, and are always underfoot, allowing the spouse no space, peace or privacy. In so doing they are more likely to alienate affections and increase the spouse's impatience.

Increased anxiety is a common occurrence in persons who have suffered mild strokes where there is an awareness that mental efficiency is reduced and there are fears of not being in control of their lives. Anxiety undermines the person's self-confidence, and the resulting feelings of inadequacy tend to make him very cautious in attempting anything new and reluctant to be left by himself.

Most stroke survivors suffer some form of depressive reaction which may be transient or become chronic. It is not surprising in view of the many frustrations, difficulties and uncertainties that have to be faced. Reduced physical or mental capacities, loss of status, job, financial insecurity and the possibility of permanent loss of independence all contribute to depression. Depressive behaviour is disturbing because it is pervasive and there is so little that family members can do to relieve it.

SPECIFIC FAMILY RELATIONSHIPS

Husband and wife

When one partner becomes incapacitated as a result of a stroke, the quality of the relationship inevitably alters. The major source of companionship and emotional support may have been lost and the psychological impairments may make it difficult to re-establish a normal marital relationship. The healthy spouse may assume the role of caretaker and at the same time be required to take over the responsibilities (financial, domestic etc.) previously managed by the other partner. Not only is the workload increased, but there are often additional expenses just when income has been reduced. Social activities decline, and friendships may dissolve. Loneliness and depressed mood may result so that it is important for the healthy spouse not to neglect their own needs, to take time to do enjoyable things, to spend time with friends, to ensure adequate diet, exercise and plenty of sleep.

A reduction in sexual expressiveness and sexual intercourse is common because of reduced libido, fear of inability to perform and fear that sexual intercourse might cause another stroke. Such anxieties are understandable but there is no reason why sexual activities cannot be resumed although physical positioning may need to be altered to accommodate physical disabilities. Sometimes specific brain lesions produce heightened sexual arousal and may result in persistent demands being made of partners. The healthy partner may also find it hard to cope with inappropriate sexual remarks, reduced social and emotional sensitivity, and paranoidal suspiciousness of fidelity.

For healthy spouses, it is difficult to mourn the partner who is still there with the familiar body, voice and ways but who is no longer the person they knew and loved. If the healthy spouse, or any family member, continues to treat the significantly changed person as they remember them, they are bound to be disappointed and frustrated. Old habits of thinking and dealing with the person will need to be relinquished and newer patterns and ways of dealing with the person developed in their place.

The patient's child or sibling

Children of a stroke person often express fear of death and concern that their behaviour may have contributed to the parent's illness. They are well aware that the illness has resulted in considerably less attention from parents than usual and that there has been a corresponding increase in responsibilities. Often they express feelings of frustration and anger that their family is different, and may be ashamed to bring friends home. They may be frightened of the parent's behaviour and may find they are competing with that parent for the other parent's attention. Parents may not have the time to be involved in school or other activities as much as they did before. Older children may act out their fears and resentments, by running away, dropping out of school, getting into trouble with the police. Children need to be reassured that they are still loved in spite of the changes that have occurred.

Siblings of younger patients have similar concerns and reactions, finding they are no longer receiving the attention or care they feel they deserve. Siblings and children benefit from information about stroke and its effects, and from opportunities to discuss their feelings and fears.

Family and friends

Family and friends who do not visit often may not be aware of the subtle difficulties the person may encounter daily. It may assist the healthy spouse if such concerns are discussed with friends since this may assist in sharing concerns and in developing new approaches to these problems.

In general, family and friends should attempt to help the person help themselves, fostering independence, and should relate to the person in the usual way. If slowness and communication difficulties are present, the person should be given time to talk or think through problems. Where there have been alterations in personality and behaviour, family and friends should be encouraged not to take remarks personally, not to provoke or argue with the individual, and not to pander to every request or be over-solicitous. It is important always to try to reduce tension.

It is important also, to highlight what the person can do rather than dwell on disabilities, and at different times to consider what the difficulties might be that may be interfering with thinking or performance.

Caring for someone who has suffered a stroke may bond a family closer together or may impose enormous burdens on the spouse and family which may tear it apart. Being informed about the effects of stroke, understanding the difficulties that might be encountered and appreciating that recovery is a slow process may help in making the necessary adjustments. Survival for caregivers requires staying with the present rather than brooding about how catastrophic the future may be, highlighting the strengths and daily achievements rather than the weaknesses, making time to care for themselves, and being wise enough to ask for help when it is needed.

CHAPTER 4

How Stroke Is Treated

Dr. Stephen Davis

While stroke remains the third most common cause of death in most Western countries after heart disease and cancer, there has been a progressive decline in the number of new strokes over the past twenty-five years. This dramatic improvement has been chiefly due to the effective diagnosis and treatment of high blood pressure and other risk factors.

RISK FACTORS AND ASSOCIATED DISEASES

Any discussion of stroke therapy must therefore emphasise the importance of stroke prevention, which involves the treatment of risk factors and warning attacks (TIAs) that often precede an established stroke.

High blood pressure (hypertension)

High blood pressure is the most important risk factor for the two common types of stroke, namely cerebral infarction (where the brain is "starved" of oxygen, usually due to blockage of blood vessels by clot) and cerebral haemorrhage (where the vessel actually ruptures, with the formation of a blood clot within the substance of the brain). Large population studies have demonstrated an increased risk of stroke among individuals with high blood pressure, particularly when moderate or severe. High blood pressure causes acceleration of "hardening of the arteries" (*atherosclerosis*), increases the tendency of small blood vessels within the brain to rupture producing cerebral haemorrhage, and leads to increased heart disease.

Many clinical trials, where the effects of treatment of high blood pressure are evaluated, have demonstrated a significant reduction in the risk of stroke when patients have effective anti-hypertensive medication. It is therefore vital to detect high blood pressure early by the use of mass screening programs, as hypertension usually produces no symptoms. Many patients with elevated blood pressure can be treated without drugs by simple measures which include weight reduction, salt restriction and a regular exercise program. If blood pressure remains elevated, drug therapy is usually necessary as well as careful follow-up by the patient's doctor. Tests are often performed in younger patients with high blood pressure, to determine whether there is a specific underlying disease causing the hypertension, such as a kidney or glandular disorder that may require specific treatment. In elderly patients with hypertension, blood pressure reduction with medication has to be performed gradually and with caution, due to the risks of confusion and fainting in this age group.

Associated heart disease

One of the most common types of stroke is caused by blood clots forming in the heart, travelling to and blocking brain arteries. In the past, rheumatic fever was a common disease, often producing abnormalities of the heart valves and irregularities of its rhythm. Fortunately, this condition is now much less common and attention has particularly focussed on the disorder termed *atrial fibrillation* where a small cardiac chamber called the atrium does not contract normally, resulting in an irregular heartbeat and an increased risk of formation of blood clots within the heart and a subsequent stroke. A number of clinical studies have indicated that blood-thinning agents (anticoagulants) are useful in the prevention of this type of stroke.

Diabetes

Diabetes is associated with a threefold increase in the risk of stroke, mainly due to acceleration of hardening of the arteries supplying the brain. The early recognition and effective control of diabetes are both desirable, although the benefits for stroke prevention are uncertain.

Smoking

It is now recognised that cigarette smoking is a very important risk factor for stroke, as well as for heart disease and disease in the peripheral blood vessels of the limbs. Smoking also increases hardening of the arteries supplying the brain as well as those within the heart, and lowers the brain's blood flow. Measures to reduce smoking in the general population will contribute to the reduction of the rate of stroke in our society.

Other risk factors

Elevation of blood fat, particularly cholesterol, is a relatively weak risk factor for stroke although more strongly associated with heart disease. Heavy alcohol intake, particularly "binge" drinking, is related to an increase in the risk of stroke. An increase in blood stickiness, particularly due to an elevation in the number of red cells in the blood increases the risk of stroke.

Although the oral contraceptive pill has been linked with stroke, it is probably a very rare cause, particularly with the introduction of the low oestrogen dosage forms. Psychological stress has not been specifically associated with increased stroke risk.

WARNING ATTACKS (TRANSIENT ISCHAEMIC ATTACKS—TIAs)

Many strokes are preceded by brief warning attacks where the patient develops transient weakness, disturbance of speech or vision, often lasting only a few minutes. Patients often consider that they are "having a stroke", but are then relieved when the symptoms resolve within a short space of time and may not seek medical advice. It is recognised that such warning attacks (TIAs) are associated with a five to tenfold increase in the stroke risk per year and they require urgent specialist investigation and treatment.

These attacks are often due to narrowing of the major arteries in the neck that supply the brain, whereby small clots or clumps of fat from the lining of the artery are carried by the flow of blood, resulting in transient blockage of the small arteries in the eye or brain. Less commonly, they are due to irregularities of the heart rhythm or abnormal heart valves.

Investigations often involve a brain scan (*Computerised Axial Tomography* or *CAT scan*) which provides the doctor with horizontal imaging "slices" through the brain, and other tests that provide information about the blood supply to the brain. The traditional x-ray of the brain's arteries is called *angiography*. This involves the injection of dye (usually via a fine tube inserted under local anaesthetic) into the artery in the groin. More recently, "non-invasive" techniques that employ sound waves (*Doppler ultrasound*) have been introduced, providing information about the moving blood cells within the arteries, as well as the vessel walls.

Treatment of TIAs

If there is severe narrowing or ulceration of the major arteries within the neck (the carotid arteries) supplying the brain, an operation called carotid endarterectomy is sometimes performed by a specialised vascular surgeon or neurosurgeon. It involves removal of the narrowed and diseased blood vessel lining in the neck. This procedure is done in order to prevent a major stroke due to formation of a large blood clot at this site, where the blood flow is typically slow and turbulent. In many patients, medical therapy with aspirin is used. The importance of aspirin in stroke prevention has been recognised in recent years. It is particularly effective, in a small dosage (half or one aspirin tablet per day), in stroke prevention in patients who have had a warning attack. Blood thinning treatment (anticoagulation) with medication called warfarin is often used in patients with a heart abnormality (such as irregular rhythm or abnormality of a heart valve) when it is considered that the patient is at risk of stroke.

The investigation and treatment of patients with warning attacks should be conducted by a medical expert in stroke prevention. This doctor may be a specialist physician, or vascular surgeon or neurologist. These clinicians have considerable experience in stroke prevention and treatment, have access to modern investigative facilities and work closely with other medical and surgical colleagues who have expertise in this area.

DIAGNOSIS AND TREATMENT OF ESTABLISHED STROKE

The doctor treating a patient with stroke has to consider five basic questions. These are:

1. Is it a true stroke or a condition mimicking stroke?

2. Is it a cerebral infarct (usually vessel blockage due to clot) or cerebral haemorrhage (blood vessel rupture)?

3. What part of the brain or specific artery is affected and what is the underlying cause?

4. Is the stroke progressing or has the patient stabilised?

5. What is the best way to prevent a further stroke?

Diseases mimicking stroke

The diagnosis of stroke is usually straightforward. Patients have a sudden or relatively sudden onset of weakness down one side of the body, disturbance of balance or speech, disturbance of sensation or vision and often drowsiness or actual loss of consciousness. Frequently, they have associated headache and sometimes have an epileptic seizure.

Other medical conditions, however, can produce precisely these same symptoms, although their treatment is quite different. These disorders include infections within the brain, certain types of brain tumour, blood clots on the surface of the brain (beneath the skull) and disturbances of the blood chemistry, particularly low blood sugar. It is now standard practice to investigate patients with stroke with a CAT scan, and often other special tests, to rule out these other diseases which often require urgent therapy.

Cerebral infarction versus cerebral haemorrhage

The distinction between cerebral infarction and haemorrhage is vital, as some patients with haemorrhages (clots within the brain) are treated by urgent surgery and some patients with infarcts are treated with blood thinning agents, which would be potentially catastrophic for those with ruptured vessels.

While patients with cerebral haemorrhage appear often more "ill" with drowsiness or coma, the reliable distinction between infarct and haemorrhage relies on the early use of CAT scanning. This test has transformed the investigation and management of stroke.

The location of stroke and the underlying cause

Using neurological examination as well as special investigations (particularly the CAT scan), doctors try to determine what part of the brain has been affected by stroke and the underlying cause. For example, language disorders which affect speech, reading and writing in a right-handed individual indicate an abnormality on the left side of the brain, whereas a right-handed patient with left-sided weakness and a peculiar unawareness of their problem would suggest a stroke affecting the right side of the brain. Strokes affecting the brain stem, the structure at the base of the brain where fibres from both halves of the brain converge and supply the spinal cord, often produce abnormalities affecting both sides of the body as well as speech and swallowing problems.

The cause of a stroke is most often determined by careful clinical examination. For example, the development of stroke in a patient with an irregular heartbeat or recent heart attack, would suggest the likelihood of a clot from the heart, which has travelled to the brain. A noise (*bruit*) heard by a doctor using a stethoscope to listen to the arteries in the neck might suggest that a narrowed blood vessel has led to a blood clot in the carotid artery, which has subsequently travelled to the arteries of the brain producing a brain infarct. The finding of severe neck stiffness in a patient who developed a sudden, devastating headache, with or without localised weakness, suggests a superficial vessel rupture on the surface of the brain, called a subarachnoid haemorrhage.

Other special tests are performed in selected cases, including angiography, Doppler ultrasound and cardiac investigations.

Treatment of the stable stroke patient

In general, patients with stroke should be admitted to a hospital facility for specialised nursing and medical care, specific investigations, physiotherapy and assessment by allied health professionals.

In the patient who is stable, initial treatment consists of skilled medical and nursing care. Patients often have difficulty swallowing and may require a feeding tube inserted via the nose and leading to the stomach (nasogastric tube) or intravenous drip. Care is taken to prevent complications in patients who are initially restricted to bed, such as pneumonia or clots in the blood vessels of the legs.

Some hospitals have designated specific wards for the care of stroke patients, whereas others have developed a specialised Stroke Service (a team which includes doctors, nurses and allied health professionals who have a specific interest in stroke and who work as a coordinated group), whereby stroke patients can be treated in various wards of the acute hospital.

Patients with stroke often have elevated blood pressure, and a stroke itself can cause further blood pressure elevation. Any reduction of blood pressure has to be performed with great caution, as this can lead to a deterioration in the patient's condition.

A coordinated rehabilitation program should be commenced at an early stage, once the patient has stabilised and investigations are completed. Physiotherapy is used to prevent complications such as pneumonia or muscle contractions, to start mobilisation and motor relearning as early as possible. The speech therapist evaluates any swallowing disorders and initiates the treatment of language difficulties (*aphasia*). The occupational therapist assesses the patient's functional impairment.

The Stroke Team usually meets on a regular basis and advises on the patient's specific rehabilitation needs. This will usually involve the transfer of a patient to a rehabilitation unit.

Treatment of the deteriorating stroke patient

Up to 30 per cent of patients with stroke continue to deteriorate after they are admitted to hospital. This includes patients with both cerebral infarction and haemorrhage and is often due to progressive swelling of the brain and elevation of pressure inside the skull.

Unfortunately, medications that reduce brain swelling in other disorders (such as brain tumors), particularly cortisone (steroids), are ineffective in patients with stroke.

Thinning of the blood with intravenous heparin (which prevents blood clotting) is often used in selected patients, particularly those with narrowed arteries within the neck, where the patient's progressive deterioration is thought to be due to further blood clots travelling to the brain. The effectiveness of this treatment remains controversial, while it is of established value in stroke prevention in those with heart abnormalities (see below).

Although surgery of the blood vessels in the neck (carotid endarterectomy) is used in selected patients as a stroke prevention measure after minor warning attacks, this treatment is rarely used in patients with completed or deteriorating strokes due to clots in the carotid arteries, as the surgery in unstable patients can cause further deterioration.

Several new therapeutic approaches are being currently evaluated in large clinical trials, aimed at limiting the consequences of stroke, and to both prevent and treat deterioration in patients once stroke has occurred. These techniques include the use of therapy to dissolve blood clots, already shown to be a valuable form of treatment in patients with heart attacks. The chief risk of this therapy is the production of cerebral haemorrhage. It is also recognised that irreversible brain damage occurs within a short time of vessel blockage and that clot-dissolving treatment, to be effective, must be used very shortly after the onset of symptoms.

Other treatments currently being explored include the use of intravenous therapy which both increases the volume of blood within the brain's arteries (with the aim of increasing brain blood flow and hence oxygen delivery to the damaged area), often combined with treatment to reduce the concentration of red blood cells in the blood. Drugs which block certain actions of the chemical calcium can expand small arteries within the brain and also reduce the consequences of brain damage. One such drug, nimodipine, has been shown to improve the outlook in patients with superficial (subarachnoid) cerebral haemorrhage, where the blood vessels often go into spasm after the initial bleed, due to the irritative effects of the blood which bathes the injured artery. This drug therapy is also being evaluated in clinical studies of other types of stroke.

Treatment of patients with progressive cerebral haemorrhage

In selected patients with cerebral haemorrhage, who have blood clots within the substance of the brain producing compression and often progressive deterioration, urgent surgery can be employed whereby the blood clot is evacuated. This is particularly important in patients with blood clots affecting the balance centre of the brain (cerebellar haemorrhage). Recent advances allow the precise localisation of blood clots within the brain and computerised placement of surgical probes (stereotactic surgery) which permit the evacuation of blood clots, with much less risk of damage to the surrounding brain. This treatment is sometimes considered in patients who progressively deteriorate under observation and where the haemorrhage is relatively superficial in the brain's substance.

Patients with superficial (subarachnoid) haemorrhage comprise a special group, the strokes often occurring in young patients and due to the development of aneurysms on the brain's arteries, which are "bubbles" that form on weak, branching points, sometimes in patients with high blood pressure. These patients are at particular risk of further catastrophic haemorrhages as well as blood vessel spasm and are usually treated by urgent surgery.

Prevention of recurrent stroke

Approximately 20 per cent of patients die from the immediate effects of the stroke, usually within a few days of admission to hospital. Surviving patients are at risk of further strokes, often more severe than the initial one.

It is therefore vital to employ stroke prevention techniques wherever possible, and this depends on an understanding of the precise cause of each patient's stroke and an understanding of their likely "natural history", that is the likelihood of further stroke in the future if that individual patient receives no specific treatment.

Patients with strokes due to a narrowed blood vessel within the neck (carotid disease) are considered for surgery if they have a severe blockage of the appropriate artery and if they make a reasonably good improvement with rehabilitation. This surgery is usually deferred for four to six weeks after the stroke, as early operation is associated with increased risk. However, when a patient has had a very minor stroke, early surgery may be performed with relative safety. Many of these patients are treated with aspirin which reduces the blood stickiness and hence the risk of recurrent clotting.

In patients with stroke due to clots from the heart, blood thinning agents that prevent clotting (anticoagulants) are often used early after the first stroke. For example, in patients with one form of grossly irregular heartbeat (atrial fibrillation), intravenous anticoagulation with heparin is often used within a day or so of the onset of the stroke, as this group of patients has up to a 20 per cent risk of a further stroke within two or three weeks of the event. Oral anticoagulation with warfarin is often continued for months or years in these patients, following the initial intravenous treatment.

Careful reduction of high blood pressure is important in stroke prevention, as is the treatment of the other risk factors considered at the beginning of this chapter. In most patients with cerebral haemorrhage, high blood pressure is the usual culprit, producing rupture of the fine deep vessels within the brain substance. Effective treatment of hypertension is therefore crucial in the prevention of further cerebral haemorrhages. Underlying abnormal blood vessels (aneurysms, or blood vessel malformations involving the arteries and veins) are sometimes delineated by blood vessel x-rays (angiography) and require specific neurosurgical treatment.

INVESTIGATION AND TREATMENT OF STROKES IN CHILDREN AND YOUNG ADULTS

Although stroke is regarded as a disease associated with advancing age, some strokes occur in children and young adults. These are often due to malformation of blood vessels within the brain, heart abnormalities or conditions causing an increased tendency for blood clotting.

This type of stroke patient requires urgent and extensive investigation for a range of relatively rare conditions, which often require specific therapy. For example, minor abnormalities of the heart valves, not obvious to clinical examination, may be diagnosed by special techniques that utilise ultrasound (soundwaves). Investigations may reveal abnormalities of the blood clotting system, where the blood has an increased stickiness or tendency to clot. Sometimes, inflammation occurs in small blood vessels within the brain and may respond to the use of anti-inflammatory agents, such as cortisone. Blood vessels in the neck can be torn due to relatively minor injuries, leading to the formation of blood clots and subsequent strokes.

Blood clots can form in the veins of the brain, termed *cerebral venous thrombosis*, particularly seen in patients with an increased tendency to blood clotting and sometimes in patients with inflammation of the paranasal sinuses or middle ear, in close proximity to the veins

73

of the brain. The diagnosis of clotting of the veins of the brain can be very difficult and early treatment with anticoagulation is of great importance.

The term "stroke", implying the "striking down" of an otherwise fit person has, in the past, implied a nihilistic approach to treatment. It has been considered that there has been no effective therapy for stroke, that patients either die or are left with catastrophic brain problems and rarely return to a productive life. This dismal view is fortunately far from the truth. The modern approach to stroke therapy emphasises prevention, early intervention and active therapy by doctors and other health professionals with a specialised interest in stroke treatment.

The treatment of risk factors and warning attacks prevents a stroke from occurring in many patients and it is hoped that the newer treatments will reduce the effects of stroke in many patients. Once a stroke has occurred, specific therapy is directed at prevention of a further attack.

Contrary to the often pessimistic view about the consequences of stroke, most patients recover and are able to return home and often to work, leading a good quality of life. This depends on early and coordinated rehabilitation.

CHAPTER 5

Rehabilitation Following Stroke

Dr. Graeme R. Penington

Rehabilitation is concerned with helping a person, disabled by whatever cause (and also his or her family), to achieve and maintain the best possible lifestyle. It is not just a matter of physiotherapy, or speech therapy, or any other individual therapy or combination, but an approach to the "whole person" in the social context. If possible, one seeks to help the person to eliminate the disability, and if that is not possible then to compensate so that the person may function optimally in every aspect of life — physically, psychologically, socially and vocationally. This extends also to the family circle, the members of which may be every bit as devastated by the stroke as the patient, and therefore unable, as individuals or as a group, to function normally.

First, a word about disability and handicap. Rehabilitation specialists generally follow the World Health Organisation in differentiating between impairment, disability and handicap. *Impairment* is used to indicate the loss of a bodily part or function, such as paralysis of a limb, loss of speech and so forth. *Disability* indicates a loss of personal function — loss of ability to dress, walk, carry on a conversation, wash the dishes and so on. *Handicap* refers to how a person functions in society, which is a much more complex matter.

Handicap is of course influenced by the disability, but also by the previous lifestyle, ability and training, by architectural barriers, and especially by attitudes — of the stroke person, of family, of those around them, of employers and sometimes of bureaucrats, legislators, lawyers or other officials. A computer programmer who loses leg function only, and has alternative means of mobility, need not have his or her vocational ability impaired at all. However, if the work premises are placed on the third floor of a building with no lift, then he or she faces a handicap. Similarly, if the employer insists on employing only able-bodied workers, or the toilet is not readily accessible to them, these are further potential handicaps. The professional dancer with the same disability, of course has a handicap, but might put previous skills to use in teaching or choreography with equal satisfaction. Many such people have met someone who assumes that loss of leg power automatically means loss of mental power also, although community attitudes to disability are slowly changing. The attitudes and actions of families can range from over-protectiveness or failure to recognise the scope of a person's ability to lack of acceptance of disability. Whatever the attitudes of others, the person's attitude to his or her changed situation will have a marked effect on the ultimate lifestyle. A positive outlook may go a long way towards overcoming obstacles, while a negative one can be inhibiting, and itself can be a major problem to be tackled.

Rehabilitation should not be seen as something that starts after medical treatment is finished. To be most effective, it starts from the time of first illness or injury, concurrently with the acute medical treatment measures, and continues until the optimum lifestyle has been achieved and will be maintained. This means that it may never actually stop, as continued vigilance may be necessary to stop deterioration in ability and activity, although the personnel involved and the type of activity will vary from time to time. After a period of intensive therapy, it is common for a person's rehabilitation to be guided by the staff of a day hospital, by a general practitioner or sometimes by the patient and family themselves. Indeed, not everyone who has a stroke will need to attend a specialised rehabilitation unit. Some need no help at all, some achieve excellent results with the help of their general practitioner and other community resources.

PROBLEMS AFTER STROKE

The problems that may need to be addressed after a stroke are many and varied, depending on the parts of the brain involved. Paralysis of an arm or leg is obvious when it occurs. Other motor (movement) problems that may occur are a loss of coordination (*ataxia*) or a loss of ability to carry out previously routine motor tasks (for example, putting on a jacket) despite being able to perform each of the individual movements (*apraxia*). Problems of balance are often associated with a cerebellar stroke.

Less obvious than motor paralysis, but nevertheless disabling, is loss of feeling in the limb. Even more disabling is loss of awareness (technically called "neglect" or "inattention") of the affected parts, or of part of the environment. A person with hemineglect, for example, may totally ignore food on one side of the plate, or consistently walk into door posts on the affected side. Loss of vision to one side (often wrongly interpreted by the patient as blindness in that eye) is common. Hearing may also be affected, but generally less commonly and less seriously.

Swallowing is affected quite commonly in the acute stage, perhaps requiring tube feeding for a time. Sometimes this problem will continue, requiring special assessment and therapy. Similarly, bowel and bladder function may need special attention.

Communication may be affected in many ways. The problem may be one of actual mechanical production of speech or writing, of reception of information, of mentally processing and storing it, of planning a response, of formulating the details of the response, or turning those details into grammatical form and directing the speech or writing mechanism to produce the sounds or writing.

Loss of intellectual, psychological and emotional functioning can be the most serious of all problems, for both patient and family, although perhaps not obvious to the casual observer. Family relationships can be severely strained as a result of the behavioural or personality change. Depression affects a large proportion of stroke sufferers, and not only as a reaction to the lost function — it is also caused specifically by the brain damage, but in either case should respond to suitable treatment. Sexual functioning can be seriously affected, although the patient and spouse will frequently not mention this unless encouraged to do so, and much can be done to help if this is the case.

In short, absolutely any aspect of life may be affected by a stroke, and most times the problems can be reduced if not completely removed by appropriate action, so it is important that patients and their families should feel free to discuss any concerns with the treating staff.

RECOVERY OF FUNCTION

Once it was thought that damaged brain had no recuperative ability, but it has been shown that new connections and pathways can develop. These new connections may or may not be useful (for example, they may encourage the development of spasticity). Rehabilitation therapy aims to encourage useful connections while inhibiting undesirable developments as far as possible.

While most spontaneous recovery of brain function occurs in the first three months after a stroke, the recovery process may actually continue for at least five years, and throughout this time can be modified by therapy. While undoubtedly early rehabilitation gives the best prospect for improvement, surprising results have been achieved by later commencement of therapy. It can be extremely difficult to predict the extent of a person's ultimate recovery after a stroke, so many experts feel that every person who survives a stroke and is conscious should have the benefit of at least some rehabilitation therapy. Unfortunately, limited health care resources usually make this impracticable, and some selection must then be made of the patients most likely to benefit. However, a person not considered suitable at one time (even after a series of reviews) may at a later date show potential and warrant review and reconsideration.

BASIC REQUIREMENTS FOR REHABILITATION

The most critical factors a rehabilitation specialist looks for in assessing a person after a stroke are the degree of alertness, and the capacity to cooperate and to learn. These do not necessarily require oral speech, but some sort of basic communication is needed, even if only by gesture or by the patient's physical response to the therapists' requests, which may be augmented by physical cues. The patient also needs some ability to concentrate and remember what has been taught (long-term memory may be intact, yet recent memory, which is critical to learning, may be severely deficient).

Without these abilities, a patient is not going to benefit from a specialised rehabilitation program. Sometimes, these abilities will not be present for some time, but return satisfactorily at a later time.

Other useful indicators are presence or recovery of control of the trunk (allowing the person to sit unsupported), some return of leg power, and control of bowel and bladder function. Loss of sensation or of spatial or bodily awareness, and persisting incontinence of bowel are adverse signs, but certainly not of themselves contraindications to admission to a rehabilitation program. Unsafe swallowing should never prevent rehabilitation, but may be a reason for referral to a centre with special expertise in that regard. Physical stamina may be compromised by coincident medical problems to such an extent that an active program is impracticable until these problems are resolved.

Lack of function in an arm, particularly at three weeks after the stroke, indicates a high probability that the arm will remain disabled to some degree, and probably to a major degree, in the long term. Fortunately, however, most activities can still be performed one handed even if adaptive aids are needed. For example, there are a significant number of one-handed musicians. Motivation to participate is important, and may be impaired by many factors which may need attention before, or concurrently with, the intensive rehabilitation therapy.

Lack of social support is definitely an adverse factor. People with a supportive spouse are far more likely to return home than those who are isolated. However, life in a nursing home may be greatly enhanced by a period of rehabilitation therapy. Any decision regarding active rehabilitation will normally be based on the totality of evidence, including the patient's wishes (if able to be ascertained), and on the availability of resources for rehabilitation.

AN OVERVIEW OF REHABILITATION

The following general description of a patient's progress through a rehabilitation program after a stroke would be fairly typical:

Having been admitted to the rehabilitation ward, the patient is visited by doctors, rehabilitation nurses and therapists of most, if not all, disciplines. They assess the patient's problems and potential, previous lifestyle and wishes for the future. Meantime the patient is getting used to the different setting, and the lifestyle in the unit, which is probably very different from that in the acute hospital ward he or she has left. For example, the emphasis is on the patients doing what they can instead of being passive recipients of attention. Most are out of bed all day, dress in everyday clothes and eat meals in a dining room. Bedpans and "bottles" are discouraged as the whole idea is to recreate normal living as far as practicable. Nevertheless, in some circumstances a patient may be discouraged from doing something that seems possible, for special therapeutic reasons.

After the assessment, all the staff sit down together to collate their information and define the major problems, long-term and short-term goals in general and specific terms, and develop plans of action for the next few weeks. The patient's wishes will have been considered in this planning and the results of the staff discussions then discussed with the patient, to ensure his or her agreement. With the patient's agreement, the family (who have usually had individual discussions with some staff already) are invited to sit down with the team to discuss the same issues (and any other queries they may have). This enables the staff to gain further background information about the patient, and the family to gain an idea of what to expect along with specific suggestions from the staff as to how family members can help.

Most therapy sessions occur on weekdays, and sometimes family members will be encouraged to attend certain sessions to learn how best to help the patient. The patient who has worked hard through the week may well need the weekend off. Nevertheless, all activities, day and night, should be consistent with the therapy plans. Outings with the family are encouraged as soon as feasible. These give a break from the routine, and an opportunity to practise newly learnt skills. Initially the outing may be a drive in a car (the staff helping the patient in and out of the car). As mobility improves, and if the home is accessible and layout and facilities suitable, visits home for a few hours, a day, overnight, then all weekend are usual.

At some stage, staff will usually visit the home to assess its accessibility and to suggest ways of making it easier for the patient to live at home (for example, adjustment to bed height or firmness, installation of "grab rails" especially in bathroom and toilet, provision of a bath seat and hand-held shower, adjustments to doorways). Many rehabilitation services have their own handyman to assist with minor alterations and installations.

At intervals during the patient's stay, progress is reviewed formally by the whole team together and problems, goals and action plans redefined. The patient and family are of course party to these reviews, whether actually present at the meetings or not.

As discharge time approaches, plans for ongoing management will be made in liaison with appropriate people and agencies. A careful follow up is most important, to ensure continued improvement, to check development of bad habits or of other problems, and to arrange review by a rehabilitation specialist, physician or neurologist if appropriate. It may be that the patient will continue to attend the unit as a day patient for some time, to continue participating in an intensive program. Attendance at a day hospital, day centre or community health centre, or a home therapy program are among other possible options. If return to work is possible, liaison with the employer and work-place visits by therapists may be helpful.

SPECIFIC PROBLEMS AND AREAS OF ACTIVITY

Motor retraining

There are a number of different approaches to therapy for impaired motor (movement) function. All aim in the long run to achieve the safest and most normal-looking pattern of arm and leg function (particularly the walking pattern) that is possible. Some emphasise special patterns of movement of the limbs and special exercises designed to restore balance, some concentrate more on sensory stimulation while others concentrate on normal patterns of movement without a lot of floor and mat exercises. Sometimes a combination of approaches is used. No one treatment approach has yet been proven to be clearly superior, as the task of proving this conclusively is particularly difficult. In most cases, it is important that the approach to movement used in the therapy department carries over into the everyday activities in the ward — for example, the method of getting into and out of the bed and chairs.

Where there is loss of sensation in a limb, or of awareness of the existence of the limb (or of spatial orientation), then special steps will be needed to protect the limb from injury as well as assisting the return of sensation and awareness. These steps may include positioning of the limb, and of the bed and chair; sometimes special techniques of skin stimulation will also be used. The family (and staff) may be asked to approach the patient only from one side, to help reinforce awareness of space on that side of the body.

A variety of walking aids are available, but many therapists try to avoid their becoming a necessity, aiming for an aid-free, normal-looking gait if possible. These aids include walking frames which require two-handed holding, four-point or three-point sticks which stand alone, and single-pointed walking sticks. If foot drop (inability to lift the foot up at the ankle) is a sufficient problem to interfere with walking, footwear may need to be modified or an orthosis (caliper, brace) provided.

Electrical treatments used in stroke rehabilitation include "functional stimulation", "biofeedback" and deep heat therapy, often in the form of ultrasound. The first is used to stimulate weak muscles, to help in maintaining their condition and to assist in their retraining by showing the patient what movements they produce (a form of biofeedback). The usual type of biofeedback machines used receive a signal from a contracting muscle, or from a pressure sensor (for example, in the shoe during gait training) and convert it into a noise or the movement of a needle (or both) so the patient perceives a response to their effort, even if the muscle contraction was too weak to produce obvious movement. Deep heat treatments may relax tight muscles allowing them to be stretched, and stimulate blood circulation and healing of damaged tissue.

The Shoulder

The shoulder will frequently give considerable problems after a stroke, and may become extremely painful, stiff or both. The shoulder joint and the surrounding tissues are particularly vulnerable to injury, the head of the arm bone (humerus) being held in place in the socket (glenoid cavity) of the shoulder blade (scapula) mainly by the muscles acting around the joint. If these are weakened, the pull of gravity can easily lead to the head of the humerus slipping out of the glenoid cavity to some degree (subluxation), stretching the sinews (ligaments and tendons) about the joint. Many people in the age group most affected by stroke already have some damage to the shoulder tissues (often without knowing it) and further stretching or tearing may lead to scarring and stiffening ("capsulitis", "rotator cuff syndrome", "supraspinatus tendonitis", "frozen shoulder"). Occasionally the whole arm may become exquisitely painful, swollen and sensitive (particularly the hand), and the skin shiny and thin. This last condition is known by various names, the commonest being "shoulder hand syndrome" and "reflex sympathetic dystrophy".

Prevention is always better than cure, and the paralysed shoulder needs special attention from the onset of the stroke. Positioning, support and movement are all important. It is particularly important *not* to pull on the affected arm (for example, in order to help the person to stand up), as this can almost be guaranteed to stretch the vulnerable tissues. Resting the arm on a tray set at the correct height and angle generally gives the best support when sitting, while various types of slings or harnesses (which grip the upper arm and exert some pull upwards) may be used when the patient is standing and walking. Harnesses generally do not actually prevent subluxation, but if correctly used may dramatically reduce the amount of pain. When capsulitis or dystrophy are developing, deep heat (usually ultrasound), skilled mobilisation, positioning, medication and occasionally injections may be used in treatment.

Spastic tightening of muscles, if unchecked, may cause joints to be drawn into deformed positions impeding function and causing pain. Heat, ice, stretching, posturing, movement, splinting, tablets, local injections, and rarely even cutting tendons or nerves may be used in treatment. Spasticity will be mentioned again when considering aftercare.

Activities of daily living

Activities of daily living, or ADL, are principally the province of occupational therapists (but not the only area in which they have expertise). Dressing, bathing, and so forth come under the heading of "personal ADL". This, together with "domestic ADL", "work ADL", "recreational ADL" and "community ADL" (travelling on public transport, shopping and so forth) will all need attention.

Where the previous way of doing a task is not possible, an alternative way can nearly always be found, either by modifying the task or the materials used (for example, velcro instead of buttons) or by providing aids to make the task easier (for example, a long handled gripper for picking things up). Assessing and relearning ADL will frequently require visits and trials in the normal surroundings at home, at work and so on. A visit to an Independent Living Centre may be warranted, to try out aids on display or receive information about other possible solutions to a problem (including the development of a special aid if no commercial aid is suitable in a particular situation).

Bowels and bladder

Anyone confined to bed, especially if not fully alert and not able to communicate readily, can develop difficulties with control of bowel and bladder. If the bowel has not opened for some days, an increasing constipation may develop, further impeding bladder control. Difficulty sitting securely on a pan toilet or commode, lack of privacy and embarrassment because of unaccustomed physical dependancy can all compound the problem.

Assuming the person is sufficiently alert and aware, sensitive nursing and use of a suitable (and suitably secure and private) commode or toilet, together with proper diet, adequate fluid and judicious use of laxatives may relieve the bowel problem. But if not, then investigation of the cause and specific therapy and a retraining program may be indicated.

Bladder problems may arise from many causes, some of which may be unrelated to the present illness (such as gynaecological or prostate gland problems) but which have made the person vulnerable. Careful investigation (which often includes measuring bladder pressures by "cystomery" or "urodynamics") will generally indicate the best therapy approach. Frequently this will involve attempting to void at regular set times, charting intake and output and possibly also the use of drugs. If the bladder has become over-stretched, it may be necessary to pass a catheter at regular intervals in addition to the above. Occasionally, the patient or spouse is taught to pass the catheter if "intermittent catheterisation" will be needed for an extended period; this is preferable to leaving a catheter in place as the latter can impede retraining and cause other complications.

Swallowing

Sometimes swallowing will be difficult or unsafe due to poor control of the muscles of the face, mouth and throat. It can be possible for food and especially fluids to "go down the wrong way" into the lungs without the person being aware, causing pneumonia.

Once a swallowing problem is suspected, expert assessment is called for. When swallowing is unsafe, it may still be possible to feed by mouth using special foods and techniques, but feeding via a tube ("naso-gastric" through the nose, "percutaneous gastrostomy" through the abdominal wall) either partly or wholly may be necessary. Restrictions on oral feeding must be strictly adhered to until retraining and reassessment indicate that the restrictions can be eased.

Communication

Communication is a complex process, involving reception of information by a variety of senses (sometimes all the senses at once), processing the information, formulating a response and then expressing this in speech, writing, body language and/or other action. The stroke may affect any of these aspects of the process.

Rarely, the power of speech may be lost irrevocably. In this case, alternative methods of communication will be explored by the speech pathologist (for example, message boards, alphabet boards and electrical communicators). When speech production is impaired but not totally lost, retraining is generally very rewarding but may take some time.

When the problem is in the processing of language and memory, then recovery may be more difficult to obtain. A careful assessment by the speech pathologist will help to define the precise problems, and indicate the best ways of approaching them. A lot of patience and encouragement (guided by the speech pathologist) by all concerned, especially by family and friends, will help. Again, recovery can continue over a long time.

Psycho-intellectual and sexual problems

These problems have been discussed elsewhere, and therefore will not be discussed here in detail. These problems can be at least as devastating to the patient and particularly to the family as are physical problems, or even more so, and require expert attention. Concentration, memory, planning and abstract thought may all be compromised, but in most cases can be improved by skilled therapy, or else compensatory techniques can be taught. Changes in mood and in control of emotions and behaviour may also occur. If these are coupled with lack of insight into the situation, then family relationships may be severely tested. Again, expert counselling and behavioural therapy have much to offer.

Depression (which may be accompanied by or be masked by an inappropriate cheerfulness or other behaviour), as indicated earlier, is commonly caused by stroke independently of any reaction to the presence of disability. It may require specific drug therapy in addition to, or rather than, counselling and psychotherapy.

"Sexuality" concerns the whole range of interpersonal relationships, and not only physical sexual intercourse. One's self-image and self-confidence are of fundamental importance in this regard. The attitude and actions of others towards one is of course also important. Apart from their effect on image, the effects of the stroke on mobility and dexterity can certainly influence interpersonal contact (including sexual performance), but normally a stroke does not directly alter the functioning of the sexual organs. A stroke should not have to affect our relationships with others, just as age alone does not alter our capacity for relationships (including sexual relationships). To be prepared to discuss concerns, and to accept expert help, is more than half the battle. Patients and their partners should feel free to approach any member of the staff of a rehabilitation unit, and be sure of an understanding and sympathetic response. If the person approached is not expert in that area, the problem will be discreetly redirected to the appropriate person.

Car driving

It must be assumed, even if not obvious, that after a stroke a person's ability to drive a car may be impaired compared to the pre-stroke ability. If the person may wish to drive, then this ability must be carefully assessed and corrective measures taken if necessary.

Sometimes, the only safe measure is to surrender the licence. In this case, it may soften the blow to consider the cost of maintaining a car, and the amount of taxi or other transport that can be bought with that amount, especially if subsidised travel (including taxi travel) is available. In the last resort, if a patient will not accept this advice, the doctor may notify the licensing authority with impunity that he or she considers a person unfit to drive, in order that the licence may be revoked.

Driving a car requires physical mobility, dexterity and stamina, concentration, alertness, forward planning ability and the capacity to make sudden and rapid decisions and physical responses under crisis situations. Emotional stability and control is also required, although experience on the roads suggests that many licensed drivers are lacking in this!

The rehabilitation team will be able to perform or arrange an assessment of driving ability. This will normally start with a medical assessment to define medical conditions that preclude driving (for example, a risk of sudden impairment of consciousness or inadequate vision). Other assessments include physical ability to enter a car and manipulate controls (which may be assisted with use of manufacturers' options, adaptive equipment or techniques) and psycho-intellectual suitability. An on-the-road test, preferably by a driving instructor experienced in disability and driving together with an occupational therapist specially trained in this area, gives a wealth of information. It may be that the person is currently unsuited, but that after passage of time or further therapy (which may include driving lessons), a re-assessment will be warranted.

AFTER DISCHARGE

When a person leaves the rehabilitation unit, however much prepared by community visits, home leaves and so forth, there is a considerable risk that function will regress unless positive steps are taken to counter this. Even if the person returns to employment and life is busy, this can still apply. As stated earlier, the functions of the nervous system can continue to change for a considerable time, and these changes need to be monitored and perhaps guided. This topic is discussed in the next section, but a few points will be mentioned at the risk of reiteration.

It is important that any person who has had a stroke be encouraged to be as active as possible and not to be overprotected, as physical activity is beneficial to both physical and mental health, and furthermore abilities learnt can easily be lost if not practised.

Medical supervision will allow monitoring of any risk factors that could predispose to further episodes of illness, and also the development of spasticity, depression (which has been found to increase in frequency and severity in the twelve months following discharge from hospital, and may well increase for even longer periods), and other problems (for example, difficulties with bladder and bowel) which may warrant review by the rehabilitation service. Ideally, all patients should be reviewed from time to time by the rehabilitation service, acting in a consultative capacity, for some years until the situation is fully stabilised.

Most people can learn to recognise adverse signs, and often learn how to modify them, which is to be encouraged. A good example is the management of spasticity.

Spasticity

Spasticity can be aggravated by anxiety or embarrassment, by inactivity, by coldness or wind, and in the case of the legs by a change in texture of the walking surface. Any irritant in the limb or its clothing may also aggravate spasticity. Possible irritants include stones in the shoes, ill-fitting shoes (fashion may need to give way to some extent to practicality), corns or callosities, infections or maceration between the toes or ingrown toenails. Ways of combating spasticity of course include avoiding the above aggravating factors where possible. The wise person takes particular care of the affected limbs and avoids tight garments or shoes, and when going to work on a cold morning dresses warmly, keeps out of the wind at the bus stop, keeps the legs moving and avoids worrying about people's reactions, so that a sudden increase in spasticity will not prevent him or her boarding the bus.

Sometimes spasticity will increase during the months after discharge from hospital despite the best of self-care, and specific therapy may be necessary. Physical therapy may help, the use of an orthosis (brace) may be indicated, antispastic drugs or local invasive treatment measures may be justified. Local treatments include injecting the nerve trunk or the "motor point" at the affected muscle to reduce its activity, or occasionally cutting the nerve; tendons may also be lengthened, divided or transplanted so as to take over the function of paralysed muscles.

The whole point of rehabilitation is to help the person and those close to them to enjoy life to the fullest possible extent. Anything that is interfering with that enjoyment, however trivial, silly or embarrassing it may seem, is worth discussing with the rehabilitation staff, as it may be possible to solve or minimise the problem.

CHAPTER 6

Leaving Hospital— What Now?

Heather Mudie and Clare Gray

On leaving hospital the stroke patient may have to contend with a variety of limitations, for the following two major reasons:

Interruption of the rehabilitation process due to financial reasons.

Private rehabilitation hospitals receive a subsidy from health insurance companies for stroke patients, which provides them with hospitalisation and rehabilitation services at top cover for up to 49 days.

After 49 days or less however, the patient may have to leave hospital before rehabilitation is completed, probably when acute nursing care is no longer required. This means that certain obstacles to independence which have the potential to respond to further treatment may still be evident.

In the public hospital system this problem is not generally an issue, as the average length of stay is not fixed by health insurance funds and the stroke patient often has the opportunity to stay for the full term of their rehabilitation.

On conclusion of inpatient rehabilitation, if there is further potential for improvement, outpatient facilities at rehabilitation hospitals, day hospitals or community health centre facilities may be utilised by the patient on request from the treating medical officer. Therapists may also set patients up with home programs, teaching families how to monitor these with the occasional outpatient check-up on progress.

Some time before leaving hospital an occupational therapist will conduct a home visit, usually with the patient present, to assess any problems with independent functioning at home. Potentially problematic areas are:

- outside surfaces and approaches to the house (for example, multiple steps)
- carpeted floor surfaces
- toilet
- shower facilities
- split level rooms
- internal staircases
- bed mobility
- inadequate seating
- kitchen.

If problems are discovered on this visit, the occupational therapist will organise modifications to be made such as installing grab rails or ramps; or teach alternative methods of performing a task to increase safety and independence in that task.

Home modifications and installation of equipment may possibly be funded by a government subsidy known as Provision of Aids to Disabled Persons (PADP) Scheme (this title varies from state to state). At the time of the home visit the occupational therapist will advise the patient about the criteria for eligibility.

Permanent residual dysfunction on conclusion of rehabilitation.

Certain types of stroke inevitably result in some degree of disability and limitation of life style, even after many months of rehabilitation. The obvious disabilities are loss of function of a leg or arm or loss of speech. Other disabilities which cause limitations to independent living are less obvious. These are:

- Loss of confidence

- Poor balance reactions

- Lack of awareness of condition

- Lack of realistic thinking

- Inability to think logically and sequentially

- Poor awareness of the affected side of the body and where it is in space

- Poor awareness of the visual field on the affected side

- Difficulty in organising garments spatially in order to put them on correctly

- Loss of the idea of what objects are used for or where certain garments are worn

- Inability to organise thinking or actions

- Inability to initiate activity

- Poor memory.

These problems will be obvious to the rehabilitation staff and prior to discharge the staff discuss with the family strategies for coping with these residual difficulties. If further instruction or counselling is necessary, the rehabilitation hospital, day hospital or health centre staff are available on appointment to provide this assistance.

Alternative accommodation

Sometimes for reasons of safety or disability, patients are no longer able to manage independently at home after a stroke and must seek alternative accommodation. There are various levels of alternative accommodation which should be thoroughly researched before the patient is re-settled to ensure that the new accommodation is personally suitable and meets all needs. The various levels are:

Retirement Village. This is especially suitable when both partners are frail but want freedom to live independent lives. The units are independent, but a trained nurse resides on the premises and call buttons are distributed throughout the unit.

Special Accommodation Houses. These are suitable for single people who need supervision and meals provided, but are independent in mobility and personal care. These places are often run by a trained nurse and allow freedom to venture out independently, but provide the security of supervision. Standards of special accommodation houses vary considerably, but a search usually reveals one suitable to personal requirements.

Hostel. This type of accommodation is similar to special accommodation housing. Some hostels are attached to nursing homes to which the residents can be transferred if deterioration of their condition occurs.

Nursing Homes. The government has laid down strict guidelines for nursing home eligibility. If considering the suitability of this type of accommodation for a severely mentally or physically disabled patient, a doctor or social worker will supply details of government guidelines.

Chronic Care Hospital Facilities. It is often possible to place severely disabled patients in the chronic or long-term care facilities of some public rehabilitation hospitals, but demand on these facilities is heavy and waiting lists are extensive.

Local councils, hospitals or church social workers will provide lists of the various accommodations within the local area.

The importance of setting goals

When adjusting to life after a stroke, it is important to set clearly defined, realistic goals in order to maximise the improvement and enjoyment of lifestyle.

Goals should be determined as a family, including the person who has had the stroke, and they should be based within the framework of the advice given by the rehabilitation team. It is vital that the family accepts the final outcome of a stroke, especially residual disability, and understands that because of permanent nerve cell destruction in areas of the brain responsible for certain functions, these functions may not recover. It is important *not* to compare one stroke with another in terms of recovery because the extent of permanent brain cell damage may be quite different from one to another.

Family support for the person who has suffered a stroke, in their attempt to become as functionally independent as possible, is vital in the early stages of re-adjustment. It is helpful for the family to develop an awareness of when and how to assist the person, allowing them the opportunity to do as much as possible for themselves without overprotecting them.

The stroke person should be encouraged by the family to resume as many former leisure pursuits as are realistically possible, or to take up new pursuits that are within their residual capabilities in order to ensure as full and enjoyable a lifestyle as possible.

Problematic daily living activities

Eating

Difficulties with eating occur for several reasons after a stroke. The most obvious problem is loss of functional use of one arm, necessitating one-handed eating. During the rehabilitation process where necessary the person will have been taught by the occupational therapist how to use the following equipment:

Rocker knife. This is a special knife designed to stabilise the food as it is cut.

Plate guard. This clips onto the edge of the plate to provide a "wall" against which the fork or spoon can stabilise food to be scooped up. Plates with "built in" lips can be purchased which serve the same purpose.

Built up cutlery. Knife, fork and spoon handles can be built up to provide a more stable grip for weak hands.

Certain strokes, such as brain stem strokes, cause paralysis of the swallowing mechanism causing problems with eating. This problem is potentially life threatening so that it is vital for the family to receive education in its management from the rehabilitation team's speech pathologist prior to discharge from hospital.

Paralysis of the facial muscles and loss of sensation on one side of the face can cause "pocketing" of food in the paralysed cheek as the patient cannot feel whether the mouth is empty or not. The speech pathologist will be able to advise on management of this problem.

Poor sitting balance creates problems with eating. Securing a good sitting position, with pillows behind the back and at the sides in the chair, prior to eating, overcomes this problem.

Visual field disturbance results in lack of attention to that part of the plate on the affected side, causing food to be left uneaten unless the patient has been trained to check for this and turn the plate around, or to turn the head to see the food on that side.

Meal preparation

Many one-handed gadgets and methods are available for meal preparation for the stroke person coping alone. The Independent Living Centre in each state, or occupational therapist at the local hospital or day centre, will be able to supply information and provide demonstrations of these gadgets and methods.

Shopping

Shopping can be a major problem for the stroke person, especially if it is not possible to drive or walk to the shops. Many supermarkets will deliver shopping from a telephone order which may overcome this problem to a great extent.

Certain strokes cause difficulty with money recognition and some stroke persons overcome this by handing their purse to the shop assistant to remove the appropriate money. This method relies very much on the honesty of the shop assistant, so a safer method may be to purchase the specially designed purse from the Low Vision Clinic which has divisions built in for the various denominations of cash and notes.

Dressing

There are two major causes of problems with dressing: *Hemiparesis* (one-sided paralysis) and *Dyspraxia*.

Hemiparesis: This leaves the stroke person with only one hand to use in dressing. During the rehabilitation process the occupational therapist will have taught one-handed dressing techniques, and discussed adaptations to clothing to enable independence in this daily activity. Some occupational therapy departments have video recordings of the techniques taught, so if the patient still needs help after discharge from hospital, borrowing a video may be beneficial.

Dyspraxia: Unfortunately, certain strokes affect the person's ability to know what certain garments are used for (for example, underpants may be placed on the head or socks on the hands by a person whose intellect is quite intact); or the ability to orientate garments spatially, so that the garments may be consistently put on upside down, inside out or back-to-front. These problems often resolve themselves while the patient is still in hospital, but if it appears that they will not be resolved, the occupational therapist will teach techniques to compensate for them. These compensatory techniques may involve education of the family, so if problems still exist after discharge further assistance can be sought by the family from the occupational therapist.

Dyspraxia may affect other areas of personal hygiene such as cleaning teeth, shaving, applying make-up and combing hair. If the family is aware that dyspraxia is a problem, constant vigilance is necessary to ensure the correct implement is used for each task, and accidents avoided that are caused by using the wrong implement (such as combing hair with lipstick, cleaning teeth with a fork or shaving with the shaver box rather than the shaver).

Incontinence

Stroke often affects the ability to control bladder and/or bowel functions. If this is a residual problem, the nursing staff of the rehabilitation unit or district nursing service will advise on equipment available for this, and the place of purchase.

Bathing

On discharge from hospital, district nursing or private nursing services can provide assistance with problems in showering or bathing which have not been able to be resolved by the occupational therapist following a home visit.

Driving

The stroke person who was driving prior to their stroke may be able to drive after the stroke providing there are no insurmountable problems. These problems are:

- Visual field disorders

- Severe cognitive problems

- Severe lack of control over right lower limb.

Residual problems such as lack of control of one arm, left lower limb or mild cognitive problems, may be controlled by driver re-education at one of the rehabilitation hospital's established centres. The occupational therapist at the local hospital or day treatment centre should be able to advise where the nearest driver re-education centre is situated. The staff at these centres will advise as to any adaptations to the car which may be necessary for safer driving.

Local councils distribute disabled parking stickers for drivers who need to avail themselves of disabled parking facilities.

Activity and movement

It is important to general health and well-being of the person following a stroke to be aware of the correct overall posture and positioning of the affected side, as the body alignment will very easily suffer as a result of uneven muscle control. Checking posture in front of the mirror helps to reinforce good symmetrical stance and movement.

While in hospital, the rehabilitation team would have provided education on caring for the hemiplegic shoulder and hand to prevent pain and swelling by correct wearing of slings, splints and positioning on pillows or armrests. It is very important to maintain these procedures on discharge from hospital, so if methods are forgotten, or pain or swelling occurs, contact the rehabilitation occupational therapist or physiotherapist for further education.

Maintaining as active a life as possible is vital also after leaving hospital to allow further improvement to occur and to encourage general total fitness. It is important to continue to transfer correctly from one place to another and use walking aids in the manner which the physiotherapists taught in hospital, and if any problem occurs in this area to seek advice from the rehabilitation physiotherapists.

Return to work

For the person who wishes to return to work after their stroke, the latter part of the rehabilitation process will involve them in a work hardening program. The occupational therapist will conduct a workplace visit to assess the demands of the person's job and a simulated job situation will then be set up in the rehabilitation centre to allow the patients to be upgraded in their work tasks to the level where they can cope easily with the demands of their job. Then the occupational therapist will negotiate their return to work with their employer. For further details about this process it is necessary to contact your local occupational therapist.

SETTING AIMS

The recovery from a stroke begins in hospital and continues long after returning home. When a stroke-affected person returns home they will need to have a positive approach and a definite plan to assist in their continued rehabilitation.

Many people who have suffered a stroke feel that they have lost control over their lives — they feel afraid and insecure. To help them regain their confidence a plan of action should be adopted so they will develop the capacity to make decisions once again. The rate of recovery varies from person to person. After they have been home for a while, spare time can be overwhelming to persons who have suffered a stroke. The progress made is often overlooked and they become depressed. Supportive and understanding people working with them will help overcome the problem of isolation and inactivity.

A daily plan of activities is a way to achieve their aims. Listing the aims can help them to communicate with others and to deal with the difficult times when discouragement creeps in — keeping in mind their abilities and disabilities since the stroke. When setting aims remember they need to be achievable and flexible.

Short-term aims may differ considerably from the long-term aims. It is most useful to set a time for completion.

The main aims to consider are: physical rehabilitation, personal, social/recreational, community/family. Activities will be necessary to reach these aims. Specific monitoring of these activities can be a way that the carer/family can see what progress has taken place and what areas need more concentration to assist with achieving these aims.

Physical rehabilitation

While in hospital the therapists will provide and set programs such as exercise, nutrition etc. that can be carried out at home.

Social/recreational

List activities the stroke-affected person may want to do, and the ones they enjoy most. Explore new and old hobbies and activities, allowing for their limitations. Travel has been made much easier since the disabled persons have been considered and services provided. Stroke Support Clubs are an excellent source of support and social outlet for the person who has suffered a stroke, as well as the carer and family.

Personal aims

It is important for the carer and family to support the stroke affected person's aims as much as possible.

Realistic aims should be set. Personal aims may range from dressing oneself to resuming driving.

Community/family

We all need to feel useful — to have an input into family life and decision making. Strategies can be developed with the entire family having an input. This is important to maintain self-esteem and develop self-respect. Stroke persons could consider becoming volunteers to assist other people who have had a stroke. Confidence can be built up by sharing experiences.

ACHIEVING AIMS

Remember when setting aims they should be evaluated regularly to ascertain the rate of achievement and to allow for adjustments to be made. One aim could be walking outside the front gate to two or three houses and return. Eventually the aim to walk around the block can be accomplished.

List long and short-term aims, planning effective ways of using their daily activities as steps to accomplish a long-term plan. Remembering the person's limitations, give ample time for the changes to take place.

Long-term aims

List long-term aims in each area: physical rehabilitation, social/recreational, personal and community/family. This can help the person to understand and

111

learn more about their present abilities. Planning long-term aims needs to be thought about carefully and each step to be taken slowly. This may apply to each area, such as joining a stroke club which comes under social, and a weekend away being recreational.

Once they have outlined their long-term aims the person can concentrate on the short-term and daily activities as these give them the realisation and experience of achievement and courage to strive on further.

Short-term aims

Daily activities are a means of measuring a person's success. This is necessary in order to obtain long-term aims. For example if their long-term aim is to help others the short-term aim may be to locate the volunteer agency working with people who have had a stroke. Long-term aim may be taking a short conducted tour, the short-term aim might be a weekend away with friends.

Undertake tasks such as wheelchair transfer at least three times a day with help from their carer. Practise the exercises the therapists have set.

Set realistic tasks and give them time to achieve their short-term aims. Take each day at a time, eventually this will lead to the achievement of their long-term aims.

Seek assistance from others if needed, alternating the more difficult unpleasant tasks with the pleasant ones. If, after much persistence, their daily activities seem to cause some concern, review the activities and break them down further to more realistic ones to achieve their short-term aim.

AIMS AND PROGRESS SHEET

Copy the Aims and Progress Sheet at the end of this section so the person can have as many charts as needed to assist in their planning. An example is included to show how to fill out the sheet.

Prepare separate sheets for each category: Physical Rehabilitation, Social/Recreational, Personal and Community/Family.

This daily activity list is important to prepare them to achieve their short-term and ultimate aims.

- Choose one long-term aim from the list. List the aim on the sheet and the date they want to achieve it by, for example, taking a short conducted tour.

- Now consider the strategy to help them achieve this aim. List the short-term aims or strategies they will use and dates for each achievement.

- Once they have their strategies clear, in order to reach their short-term aim, write it in "activities planned".

Day to day planning

To record their aims and planned activities they need to list the activities that they have performed and achieved, the date and their comments. Continue this process until they have reached their long-term aims. It is easy to write down planned activities but quite another thing to carry them out as they have been outlined on paper. A black or white board may be useful to record daily activities.

- Note an hour-by-hour plan of what they would like to achieve in one day. Writing down a plan can be very helpful, recognising the importance of preparing a list regardless of whether they actually carry out the plan. The carer or a member of the family could help if writing is difficult.

- Record how they passed each hour during the day. What was actually achieved may have been quite different from their plans. List every activity even if it was "staring into space".

- Evaluate these activities. Each evening ask them which activity gave enjoyment and the feeling of accomplishment. When evaluating it is important to examine why things did not work out. Look at what happened and what caused it not to work. It's not a failure — it is an opportunity to learn more about themselves and helps to determine where they may need assistance.

It is important for the carer to set aside time for themselves. Major changes to both the lives of the stroke person and the carer/family are being experienced. The daily activity list can be a way to assist both by easing some of the load of new responsibilities. The activity lists should be prepared by both as this will provide support and help avoid any misunderstandings.

Often the carer is the one who feels the most anguish after their loved one has had a stroke. It is important that the carer does not give up all outside interests. These can be included in the short-term aims list. Plan to resume most outside activities as soon as possible — carers need space and time to recharge their batteries. Looking after your health is also important, this is one way to achieve this.

SOLVING PROBLEMS

It is very important for the person to concentrate on what they can do, not what they cannot do. The acceptance of limitations is most important in order to avoid complicating problems.

Everyone is confronted with obstacles, conflicts and problems. Developing a technique for solving problems is part of maturity. People experience stressful periods in their lives, and solving these problems may mean discovering new methods as the old usual way may no longer be suitable.

Stress can make the smallest problem overwhelming. It is impossible to know what problems may occur on returning home. Therefore, the carer/family must be flexible and resolve these problems one at a time when they occur.

Steps to follow when problem solving

- Recognise the problem. It may be uncomfortable facing problems before they get out of hand but dealing with problems in the earlier stages will often lessen the stress. Sometimes problems will solve themselves, but they can worsen if left too long.

- Identify the problem. Discuss it with others around, then write it down. This can help identify and solve the problem. It may need a simple change to solve it. For example, the person may have walked with more confidence while in hospital.

- Document the person's feelings when confronted with the problem. For example, the person may say — "I am cross because I need someone near me when walking around home. I am frustrated because I want to be able to walk as I did before the stroke."

- Identify the problem and possible causes. Identifying the problem will help determine why it has happened. This will help analyse the person's behaviour. For example, the person may say: "Why am I needing someone near me when walking? I do not seem to be concentrating, and I could be trying to achieve my aim too quickly."

- A person has to decide on what they want to achieve. For example, "I want to be more independent and have my confidence back." The similarities are the same between solving problems and setting the aims. The setting of aims covers a longer life plan. The major problems are solved by using a more detailed technique.

- List all the ways you can help to ovecome some minor problems that have occurred. Write down everything that comes to mind, even things that may sound silly. Identify as many solutions as possible, work on them one at a time. Review the solution list frequently, make adjustment where necessary.

- Evaluate the plan and results. Did it work? Reward the person! If the problem still exists, try other ideas until a solution is found.

- It is advisable to follow simple steps to resolve problems, although it may be tedious and time consuming. Taking short-cuts may hinder the process. Try to follow the procedure outlined above.

FAMILY PROBLEMS

It is inevitable that families experience many problems as a result of a stroke. Problems need to be confronted one at a time. Solving the problems which are causing stress should be a group effort. Making mistakes is part of the learning process.

Counselling for families may assist everyone to learn new skills in listening, understanding, and the importance of expressing needs and thoughts. If communication problems are being experienced it is advisable to seek assistance from a professional.

Information on services in the community who provide counselling can be obtained by contacting any of the support services listed in this chapter.

PHILOSOPHY OF STROKE SUPPORT GROUPS

Stroke support clubs provide companionship and social support for individuals who have suffered a stroke. Their carer/families and friends can also share experiences. The development of communication links with people who understand the implications of life after a stroke provides comfort to many who have felt isolated. Many lose friends, visitors become rare in many cases. The stroke clubs compensate for friends lost as new friends are made.

Meeting on a regular basis helps to restore lost confidence, and is an opportunity to meet others with limitations to their lives as a result of a stroke. The sharing of experiences often helps to solve each other's problems. Everyday living skills are learned day by day. As a problem is confronted, one can work around it in time. The sharing of these experiences may assist someone later.

Support groups are a way to help the family to cope. They also help the person who has had a stroke to realign their purpose in life and make the best of each day and to achieve personal objectives.

STROKE SUPPORT SCHEME

This scheme provides assistance on a one-to-one basis using trained volunteers to aid the person who has had a stroke. The role of the volunteer is to develop a supportive relationship with a person affected by a stroke, to work with them on whatever special need is identified, and to provide encouragement to regain confidence and independence.

SUPPORT SERVICES

- Australian Brain Foundation
  616 Riversdale Road
  Camberwell Vic. 3124
  Tel: (03) 882 2203/(008) 33 3469 for telephone counselling, information and referral (Outreach)

- Stroke Support Group in your area

- The Home and Community Care Coordinator at your local council

- Neighbourhood House

- Local Community Health Centres

- Citizens' Advice Bureau

- Life Line

- Disability Resources Centre

- Rehabilitation Geriatric Centre

- District Nursing Services

- Independent Living Centres

- Do care (Victoria only).

EXAMPLE OF AIMS AND PROGRESS SHEET

AIMS:

Today's Date: ....1/3/90..

LONG-TERM AIM: ....Walk to the shopping centre......

....

Complete by ....5/6/90..................................

SHORT-TERM AIMS:

1) ...Walk in the house unaided..................................

2) ...Walk up and down steps...................................

3) ...Walk down the street two houses......................

4) ...Walk down to end of street.............................

Completed ...20/5/90...

STRATEGIES OF ACTIVITIES PLANNED:

..Walk with my spouse, friend or volunteer....................

..Walk with the therapist..

..Practise exercises to music with help of a volunteer......

....

....

PROGRESS OF ACTIVITIES:

PROGRESS/SETBACK	COMMENTS	DATE

1.

Walked around house unaided. Working on lifting leg.   4.3.90

2.

Slipped and fell.   Too eager!   10.3.90

3.

Practised walking down street.   Watching balance.

                                                                15.4.90

4.

5.

6.

....

....

....

....

....

....

AIMS AND PROGRESS SHEET

AIMS:

Today's Date: .... / .... / ....

LONG-TERM AIM: ....

....

Completed by ...... / ... / ......

SHORT TERM AIMS:

1) ....

2) ....

3) ....

4) ....

Completed ...... / ... / ......

STRATEGIES OF ACTIVITIES PLANNED:

....

....

....

....

....

....

PROGRESS OF ACTIVITIES:

PROGRESS/SETBACK	COMMENTS	DATE

1.

2.

3.

4.

5.

6.

....

....

....

....

....

....

....

....

CHAPTER 7

Preventing Stroke

Marilyn Collins

As discussed in Chapter 1, we can see that most strokes occur because of narrowing and clogging of arteries in the neck or brain. This narrowing and clogging of arteries occurs over a period of time and is known as artery disease (*Atherosclerosis*). (See Figure 12.)

Artery disease is a condition where fatty and fibre-like material builds up in patches inside the artery wall. As this develops, the vessels become narrower and less elastic. This condition can build up to clog the arteries and cut off the blood supply to a vital area. If the arteries leading to the heart are blocked this causes *heart attack*. If the arteries leading to the brain are blocked this causes a *stroke*.

A newborn infant has no artery disease, however this condition starts to develop early in childhood. It is believed that the development rate is affected mainly by:

- Diet

- Smoking

- High blood pressure.

The connection between high blood pressure and atherosclerosis is like the "chicken and the egg" argument — the presence of high blood pressure can lead to atherosclerosis and atherosclerosis can lead to high blood pressure.

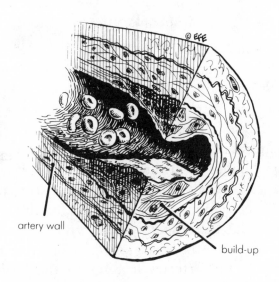

Figure 12 Artery showing artery disease (atherosclerosis)

In at least half of all stroke persons the reason why the arteries have become diseased or damaged in the first place is because people have been exposed to high blood pressure, in addition to lifestyle factors and heredity (we cannot choose our parents). Sometimes heredity is related more to lifestyle and habits shared by families and is not always genetic.

HIGH BLOOD PRESSURE

The presence of high blood pressure in men and women increases the risk of stroke and reduces life expectancy. High blood pressure is associated with high fat and salt diet, heavy alcohol intake, lack of exercise, obesity and smoking. It can be controlled through exercise and diet, though some people will also require medication. Once blood pressure is controlled it is no longer a health risk.

SMOKING

Most people are aware of the risk of lung cancer if they smoke. However, people are not generally aware that those who smoke increase their chances of having a stroke six times more than a non-smoker. *There is no safe level of smoking.*

OTHER RISK FACTORS

• High fat and salt diet

- Excess alcohol
- Lack of exercise
- Obesity
- Stress
- Heredity.

We cannot control our heredity but we can reduce our chances of developing a stroke by controlling some of the other factors which lead to stroke. These factors are often linked so much that one causes another and so on. The chart on the next page shows "reasons" for some factors linked to the development of a stroke.

The chart shows us that there are four major aspects of our lifestyle that can lead to high blood pressure, atherosclerosis, obesity and many other health problems including stroke.

Diet: A diet high in fat and salt; drinking too much alcohol leads to health problems.

Smoking: There is no safe level of smoking.

Unmanaged stress: This can lead to many health and psychosocial problems including eating problems, drinking too much alcohol and inability to stop smoking.

Lack of exercise: This increases the chance of becoming overweight, becoming lethargic, feeling bored and (for smokers) smoking more cigarettes.

127

STROKE RISK FACTORS

Factor	Reasons
Atherosclerosis	• high fat intake • high blood pressure • smoking
High blood pressure	• high fat intake • excess salt intake • alcohol consumption • overweight • no exercise • unmanaged stress • heredity
Smoking	• started when young, often due to peer pressure and advertising • once addicted then craving — a need to smoke • habit — something to do with the hands • social — joining in with others who smoke • when feeling stressed
High fat and salt intake	• choosing the wrong foods • eating too many foods • don't know which foods are high in fat and salt • don't know how to substitute low fat for high fat • don't know how to enhance flavour of foods without adding salt • eat too much when feeling depressed, bored, stressed

No exercise	• watch TV for relaxation • don't make time • exercise is tiring • prefer a drink and a smoke for relaxation
Obesity	• eating too much • eating wrong type of foods • no exercise

STRESS

Stress is part of everyday living, some people are able to cope with more stress than others. What is perceived as stressful to one person may not be stressful to another person. Stress does not cause stroke or heart disease but *unmanaged stress* may lead to some people drinking too much alcohol, overeating, smoking, not exercising, sleeping poorly and so on. This can lead to a "catch 22" situation where an individual seeks refuge for their stress in alcohol, smoking, and eating, and feels constantly lethargic, sometimes exhausted and so takes little exercise. We have all recognised some of the above in ourselves or someone we know.

So where do you go from here? Having read this, you might think that there are some unhealthy aspects to your lifestyle that you would like to change but where do you start?

First identify the areas of your lifestyle you want to change, then list the goals you want to achieve. Be realistic, do not try to change too many aspects of your lifestyle too quickly, try one goal at a time.

ARE YOU AT RISK?

Try this self assessment stroke risk chart, it may help you to identify areas where you can modify or change your lifestyle — then set yourself realistic goals.

Risk factors for stroke are factors that can accelerate development of blood vessel disease and may place you at risk of having a stroke. Assessment of risk does not determine whether you will develop blood vessel disease and stroke but it can indicate whether it is likely to occur.

- Identify areas of high risk

- Can you name some changes to reduce your risk?

- Set yourself goals — but be realistic, try one goal at a time!

CHANGING TO A HEALTHY LIFESTYLE

Making changes to your diet, drinking habits and smoking can sometimes be difficult. Some people have found success by taking up exercise first; it is also an excellent form of stress management.

Benefits of exercise

- Reduces stress

- Increases stamina

- Controls weight

SELF ASSESSMENT LIFESTYLE CHART

Risk factors	0	1	2	Score
Blood pressure	Low or normal	Raised or don't know	High	
Smoking	Non-smoker	15 or less per day	Over 15 per day	
Blood cholesterol	Below average	Average or don't know	Above average	
Weight	Normal	Overweight	Obese	
Exercise	Very active most days	Very active once or twice a week	Inactive	
Diabetes	None known	Family history of diabetes	Diabetic	
Behaviour	Easy going	Often hurried, anxious, intolerant	Always hurried, competitive, intolerant	
Heart disease	Not known	Family history	Have heart disease	
Family history	No stroke before 65	Stroke before age 55	—	
Age	Under 40	40–55	Over 55	

How do you rate?
0–3   Low risk
4–6   Moderate
7–10 High risk
11+   Very high

Total score rate?

131

- Can lower blood pressure
- Helps reduce stroke risk and many other diseases.

Exercise tips

Daily activities

- Use stairs instead of lifts
- Walk briskly to train station or bus stop
- Park your car further away from your workplace or supermarket
- Stand up and stretch arms and legs while talking on the telephone
- Tighten your stomach and leg muscles while standing
- Walk to your local shop instead of driving
- Gardening

Activities — 3 times weekly

- Brisk walking for 30 minutes
- Cycling for 20–30 minutes
- Swimming for 20–30 minutes
- Racquet sports such as tennis, badminton, etc. 30–60 minutes
- Jogging, skipping 20–30 minutes.

Remember to start slowly and gradually build up your activity levels. Brisk walking and swimming are still excellent and safe exercise choices.

Benefits of a healthy diet

- Helps control weight

- Lowers blood cholesterol levels

- Can lower blood pressure

- Helps reduce stroke risk and many other diseases

Tips to reduce fat in diet

- Cut fat off meat before cooking

- Remove skin and fat from chicken

- Choose meat which is not marbled with fat

- Avoid fatty take-aways foods, especially deep fried

- Avoid between-meal snacks of biscuits, crackers, chocolate, cakes etc. Try celery, carrot sticks or drink a glass of water

- Try low fat milk instead of full cream milk

- Reduce fats and oils used in cooking.

Tips to reduce salt in diet

- Reduce intake of salty foods such as salted snack foods, pickles, commercial sauces, salted meats, foods containing MSG

133

- Choose low salt packaged foods and those labelled no added salt

- Add no salt at the table or in cooking — substitute with herbs, spices and lemon juice.

Tips to lower alcohol intake

Recommended guidelines for alcohol consumption are 3–4 standard drinks daily for men and 2 for women.

- Drink a glass of water or non-alcoholic beverage between each glass of alcohol when attending social events

- If you have an alcoholic drink on returning home from work substitute with a non-alcoholic beverage

- If you drink wine with meals try drinking water between glasses of wine

- Avoid binge drinking.

The healthy diet

A healthy diet will include a variety of foods. The healthy diet pyramid of the Australian Nutrition Foundation provides you with a guideline — are the preparations of food in your diet similar to the healthy diet pyramid? If not try to switch your diet around so that you follow the healthy diet pyramid.

HEALTHY DIET PYRAMID

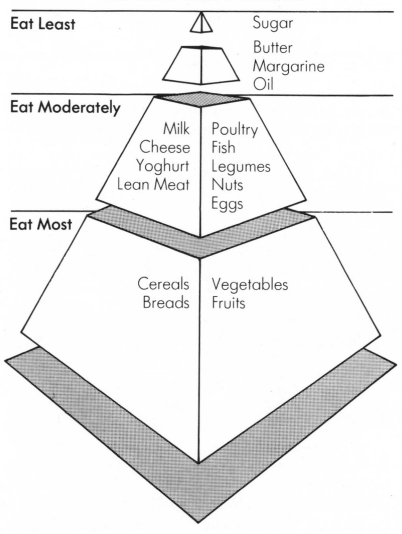

Eat Least

Sugar

Butter
Margarine
Oil

Eat Moderately

Milk
Cheese
Yoghurt
Lean Meat

Poultry
Fish
Legumes
Nuts
Eggs

Eat Most

Cereals
Breads

Vegetables
Fruits

Benefits of giving up smoking

- Feel healthier and enjoy easier breathing
- Suffer fewer colds, flu, coughs and sore throats
- Appreciate the taste of food and drink more
- Improve the health of children and others living with you
- No lingering smell on hair, clothes, breath
- No stained teeth or fingers
- Won't pollute rooms with stale tobacco, dirty ashtrays
- Save money
- Reduce stroke risk and other diseases such as lung cancer, coronary heart disease, bronchitis, and emphysema.

Tips for quitting

- Stop completely — don't cut down
- Enlist support from family, friends and work mates
- Use non-smoking areas in public places and public transport
- Remove all ashtrays
- Place the money normally spent on cigarettes aside and save up to reward yourself with something — new clothes, a night out, sporting equipment

- Have pieces of carrot, celery, fruit and vegetables chopped in a container in your refrigerator and when the urge to smoke strikes try eating these instead

- Drink a glass of water or brush your teeth

- Go for walks, take up exercise

- Try relaxation techniques

- For the first few weeks avoid situations where you might be tempted (for example, at the club, pub, with smoking friends at social functions), especially when drinking alcohol

- Drink fruit juices instead of coffee — some people find that they associate drinking coffee with smoking a cigarette.

STRESS MANAGEMENT

Many people cope with stress by overeating, smoking, drinking alcohol and sometimes taking drugs. We need to learn to manage our stress in a healthy way. There are a variety of ways this can be done through relaxation techniques, time management, assertiveness training, effective problem solving and of course, through exercise. There are many books and tapes on the subject of stress management available widely from bookstores.

Stress management and assertiveness skills training courses are conducted by a number of organisations including many community health centres, hospitals and adult education centres. Check your local telephone directory or contact your local community health centre to find out what is available in your local community.

Remember — to reduce your risk of developing a stroke, follow a healthy lifestyle:

- Be a non-smoker

- Eat a healthy diet

- Exercise regularly

- See your doctor regularly for a medical check-up including blood pressure measurement.

The Feldenkrais Method in the Treatment of Strokes

Elizabeth Beringer

Recent discoveries and developments in the movement sciences offer new help for the person recovering from a stroke. The Feldenkrais® Method is one such approach that offers an effective avenue for continued improvement after a stroke.

When the stroke itself is over the brain works actively to heal the injury. Even though many neural pathways may have been damaged the brain begins immediately to form new connections. Learning in general and particularly learning through movement helps to stimulate the brain's activity and to facilitate the formation of new pathways. This is why doctors will often recommend that someone recovering from a stroke try learning a skill that they *hadn't* known previously or something that they hadn't done for a long time. New learning is particularly conducive to the formation of new neurological connections.

A common misconception is that recovery stops a year after a stroke has occurred. In fact it is very difficult for doctors to predict after a stroke exactly what effect the damage will have on a particular person's life and abilities. There are so many different factors involved and recovery can sometimes take place through unexpected channels. A women who lost the ability to control grasping with her left hand recovered this ability while horseback riding. The stroke in which her movement was impaired occurred ten years previously, but she had not been horseback riding since she was a child. This is an example of how unusual types of movement activities can stimulate and re-educate the brain. Of course many people who suffer from a stroke will not be able to go horseback riding. However, even with severe strokes there is always some avenue through which a person can learn.

This is how the Feldenkrais Method can be helpful. The Method uses movements based on functional and developmental principles to help re-educate a person recovering from an injury such as a stroke. The Feldenkrais approach utilizes the kind of learning that takes place in children, when enjoyment, investigation and variety were all natural components of the educational process. The Method is taught through group classes, tapes or through individualized sessions. In order for an individual to learn new abilities they need to be challenged, yet this needs to go on in a supportive environment where they can be successful. For this reason the learning situations are always structured so that each person can learn at his or her own pace.

In classes or when doing tapes the student is led through gentle guided movement sequences. These are not exercises in the conventional sense, but carefully constructed exercise sequences that improve one's ability to perform important movements of daily life. A wide variety of different types of movements and functional themes are utilized in order to stimulate improvement and learning in many different areas. Benefits such as increased flexibility, ease and improved function can usually be experienced immediately. One can also go to a Feldenkrais teacher for individualized sessions. These sessions focus on the specific needs of the individual and include a hands-on approach to the learning process where the person is passively led through different movement patterns.

The Feldenkrais Method is named after the Israeli scientist Moshe Feldenkrais. He developed the Method out of his background in physics, anatomy, psychology and the martial art of judo. Since he first began actively teaching the Method outside of Israel, only twenty years ago, it has gained worldwide acclaim. The Method has a wide range of applications. It has benefited those with movement problems related to neurological or orthopedic difficulties as well as people simply wishing to move more easily and function more efficiently. This approach has been particularly useful for those recovering from a stroke because of its emphasis upon movement re-education.

CHAPTER 8

A Naturopathic Perspective

Marcus Laux, N.D.

As a naturopathic physician with a family practice in a densely populated urban area, a portion of my work includes the diagnosis and treatment of cerebrovascular accidents, strokes and transient ischaemic attacks.

I believe the treatment of a stroke patient is best served when a "health team" is actively involved in the recovery process. The "health team" approach is presently employed in several countries, with remarkable success. This more complete form of health care blends the best of current orthodox medicine with the best of traditional, natural therapies.

The primary goal of the naturopathic physician is to provide the safest non-harmful treatment that brings about the most rapid and effective healing. The patient's life can be saved by high-tech intervention, but the will to live and actual recovery process are best served when the whole person is considered and attended to. In the case of a stroke, as with many other accidents and illnesses, accurate assessment and timely treatment is imperative.

First intervention for stroke should be with the orthodox medical doctor or osteopathic physician. They are the best trained, with the technology needed for rapid diagnosis and life-saving treatment for this condition. When seconds count, this is where a stroke patient belongs. The primary concern is saving a life and minimizing real and potential brain damage. After the patient is stabilized, along with appropriate monitoring, the "complementary" therapy should be initiated. Simply put, the treatment involves caring for mind, body and soul.

An effective "health team" scenario would be as follows: A severely impaired stroke patient is brought to the hospital in critical condition. Powerful drugs and/or surgical intervention may save the patient's life and at least minimize the potential of further compromise.

Once stabilized, the patient then receives acupuncture, designed to help regain speech, memory, and the use of limbs. Massage is utilized to bring awareness to the sensory nerves; a form of biofeedback. Massage will also increase circulation, ease pain, provide passive exercise, and promote overall health.

Homeopathic and botanical remedies are employed to help normalize function, reverse any damage, and speed recovery. An individualized diet is also observed to maximize recovery and help the body heal. Special attention is given to the mental, emotional and spiritual needs of the patient. Stories are read to the patient, or he or she can read to themselves if able. The patient's room is a nurturing environment, personalized with objects from home, with sunlight pouring in through the window and soft, pleasant music playing in the background.

Support and comfort, coupled with appropriately challenging rehabilitation, mesh together for a cooperative and successful recovery and retraining.

By training and in practice, Doctors of Naturopathic Medicine are eclectic. That is, they select their therapies from a wide array of natural modalities. The treatment plan for a specific patient will be culled from this spectrum, in the combination deemed most suitable and appropriate for that patient's current symptom picture and diagnosis. The choices may include homeopathy, botanical remedies, acupuncture, prescriptive medicines, physical medicine, or any combination thereof.

Physical therapy and nutrition, as outlined in previous chapters, are integral parts of a recovery plan. The chapter on prevention is a basic blueprint for a healthy lifestyle for a stroke patient (not to mention anyone interested in improving overall health).

A naturopathic physician will place great emphasis on lifestyle patterns as they relate to prevention and therapeutics. This is the bedrock foundation for a healthy, long life with minimal distress and disease. It entails the judicious use and balance of:

- breathing pure air
- drinking pure water
- obtaining adequate sunshine
- restful, regular and adequate sleep
- maintaining proper elimination
- performing an exercise which is appropriate
- living with satisfying relationships
- spiritual practices and faith.

These elements in combination help us heal and live well. Though they are mostly self-evident, perhaps some edification regarding sunshine and spiritual practices is warranted.

Sunshine is not our enemy. Too much exposure is a problem, as is true with any excess. Sunshine has very positive effects on our glandular system and hormones, provides certain vitamins and minerals, increases metabolism, and lifts the spirits. The gradual lengthening of exposure time over several weeks is prudent to avoid sunburn, working up to a maximum of 20 minutes per day, partially clothed, avoiding the peak hours of 11:00 a.m. to 2:00 p.m., and removing any eyeware. Even if the patient only receives facial exposure, it can be of benefit.

Spiritual practice relates to prayer, church, meditation, yoga, or a walk in nature. These processes can help allay distress and quiet the mind, and also heighten awareness of the inexplicable connection with the life source. I believe this does improve our health and our quality of life, and suggest planning regularly scheduled times to get the most benefit. Attending to spiritual needs, though often overlooked in medical treatment and eclipsed by the more insistent demands of our modern lifestyle, is as important to our welfare as eating or sleeping.

Along with physical therapy, other forms of "body-work" are recommended. There are numerous variations and styles, but the intention of all bodywork is the same: restore normal functioning and improve overall health, thus bringing the patient back into "balance." The form of bodywork to be selected will be determined by factors including the patient's age, history, and severity of problems. The choices include massage, shiatsu, naturopathy, chiropractics, reiki, Trager, acupressure, and many others. When selecting a bodywork practitioner, it is essential to consider whether they are: 1) qualified in their field; 2) qualified to work with the condition to be treated; and 3) easy to communicate with (establishing a good rapport between the practitioner and the patient and/or the patient's caretaker is not to be minimized).

"Bodywork" in general, and massage specifically, can be a big plus in recovery. It has been demonstrated to have many positive physiologic effects. Besides usually feeling wonderful (no small benefit), it can stimulate growth hormone-like substances and thyroid hormone activity (i.e., it can increase metabolism and anabolic processes). Bodywork enhances repair, improves circulation, and expedites lymph drainage and other detoxification pathways. All of this and much more is the powerful effect of simple human hands applied with care and compassion. Low-tech at its best!

Several other categories are worth employing on a "multi-factorial risk-intervention" program. Acupuncture and homeopathy are both energetic medical modalities which can be very valuable. "Energetic medicines" work at the level of the body's subtle "life force." When this force is disrupted, as it would be in the case of a stroke, gentle repair is often the result of these two healing arts. Your local acupuncturist or homeopath can give further explanation of their skills and their specific appropriateness to a particular case. They may be used separately or in concert effectively.

DIET

As stated earlier, nutrition is a basic tenet for optimum, vibrant health. Alan Gaby, M.D. once summed it up nicely: "Your medicine should come from the farm, not the pharmacy." In the Orient, it is known that food and medicine are from the same source; with that in mind, let us consider diet as serious a tool as the prescription pad.

My personal qualifications of the chart on page 135 of the "Nutrition" chapter are as follows:

Eat most: vegetables
(in order) cereals (whole grains)
bread (whole grain)
fruit (seasonal)

Eat moderately: legumes
(in order) nuts
fish
poultry
eggs

Eat modestly: lean meats
(in order) yogurt
cheese (real) (if desired)

Eat least: sugar—no refined.
Substitute: Sucanat
butter—better than margarine.
Substitute: Ghee
margarine—not recommended ever
milk—only use raw fresh milk, and
only if desired
(not recommended)

> oil—olive, sesame, canola—
> use very sparingly

Some of your diet should be raw (one-third to one-half), while the balance should be cooked—steamed, baked, broiled, poached; *never* fried (my one "never").

Fresh, organic foods are superior to commercial foodstuffs.

SUPPLEMENTS

Inclusive with diet, supplements play a very important role in health care management. Sources of supplements can be plants, animals, food concentrates, isolated vitamins, minerals, and microbial products. They each have properties which help the body function normally, or perhaps enrich it to optimal functioning. These properties allow proper tonification and stimulation of the immune system, as needed, orchestrating repair and damage control. They also provide many needed catalysts and co-factors for improved oxygen-carrying capacity of the blood, causing an increase in energy and well-being. They can provide building material and the energy-enhancers to get the repair accomplished.

The importance of supplementation has been sadly lacking in the orthodox medical model. Fortunately, these days the media have been focusing on nutrition and supplementation for ever-widening benefits: anti-carcinogens, the prevention of neural tube defects in the fetus, prevention and correction of osteoporosis, goiter, rickets, anemia, hypoglycemia, wound healing...and the list continues to grow. I wholeheartedly support this new era which is upon us of food and supplementation first, then drugs later if needed. These natural substances have evolved on this planet along with us and provide crucial elements for our very existence. If we are well-nourished with adequate nutrient supplies, many health problems need never find expression; we are then naturally immune. Disease is a lack of harmony. The disease state is an expression of an imbalanced life force. Often, this can be corrected with therapeutic supplementation which is predominantly much less expensive and less harmful than drug therapy. A person is rarely ill because they have a drug deficiency, but quite often their health is impaired because of inadequate nutrient levels precipitated by poor lifestyle, diet, environmental pollution, and stress.

Strokes have two general categorizations. They are either an obstruction type or they are caused by a blood vessel rupture. Their therapy, in terms of supplementation, will also be divided into these two classifications:

Cerebral Infarction (obstruction type)
- Proteolytic Enzymes—help clean up debris and improve impaired circulation
    1. Bromelain and Papain
    2. Tyler Encapsulations—plant enzymes
- Niacin (B_3)—increase peripheral circulation, dilating
- Ginkgo Biloba
    1. Enzymatic Therapy—ginkgo phytosome; or
    2. 50:1 concentrate with 24% ginkgosides

- Lemon Juice—blood thinning capacity
- Garlic—blood thinning and anti-coagulation effect
- Willow Bark—blood thinning capacity
- Vitamin E and Selenium—antioxidants, support blood quality
- Chlorophyll—detoxifier, blood purifier, rebuilder
- Flax Seed Oil—Prostaglandin stabilizing, anticoagulant properties
- Adaptogenic Herbal Formula—increases oxygen-carrying capacity of blood; improves stress adaptation, increases body's ability to deal with increased metabolic stress
- Alterative Herbal Formula—helps clean and purify blood system

Cerebral Hemmorhage (blood vessel rupture)
- Vitamin K—helps blood clot. Short-term use initially, *only* with your practitioner's guidance
- Chlorophyll—blood purifier, detoxifier, rebuilder
- Vitamin C (esterified vitamin C)—*used by the immune system,* detoxifier, connective tissue repair
- Bioflavinoids (active, undiluted)—works with vitamin C to stabilize tissue membranes
- Crategus *Oxycantha* Extract (Scientific Botanicals)—stabilizes connective tissue membranes
- Proteolytic Enzymes—help clean up debris and improve impaired circulation
    1. Bromelain and Papain
    2. Tyler Encapsulations—plant enzymes
- Antioxidant Formula—decreases free radical damage from low oxygen content and helps stabilize

- Adaptogenic Herbal Formula—increases oxygen-carrying capacity of blood; improves stress adaptation, increases body's ability to deal with increased metabolic stress
- Mineral Complex (especially Mg/Ca/K)—prevents *vasospasms*

The Oriental patent medicines can be quite effective when used appropriately, and can be used with either type, in general. (Some formulas are manufactured by American companies with greater quality control.) Your best strategy is to seek out a competent naturopathic physician (N.D.), osteopath (O.M.D.), or licensed acupuncturist (L.Ac.) who is familiar with this modality. Some possible choices, depending on the circumstances, are as follows:

- Yan Shen Jai Jao Wan—to be taken immediately
- Mao Dung Ching capsules—more for embolic type
- Ren Shen Zai Zao Wan—recovery from brain impairment
- Tsai Tsao Wan—similar to above
- Cir-Q (Health Concerns)—excellent formula based on classic prescription "Yen Ling Tang"
- Bojenmi Chinese Tea—said to improve nutrient absorption; reputed to remove arteriosclerotic plaques from the blood vessels

Please note that supplement dosages are not given. This is intentional; the patient is urged to develop a relationship with the complementary health care provider, to tailor an individual program geared for the patient's specific needs. The practitioner needs to be fully informed of all other therapies, health history, etc. before a safe, appropriate and effective protocol can be initiated. Other medications must also be considered to avoid possible interactions.

Other therapies which may be considered or recommended during convalescence:

1. Cranial Manipulative Techniques
   These physical medicine maneuvers often can return normal functioning to the cranial circulatory system by freeing cranial suture dysarticulation. The work is often subtle and refined, with possible relief of internal pressures, thus normalizing local and systemic functioning and speeding up the healing process.

2. Chelation Therapy
   My patients have highly recommended this therapy for a myriad of circulatory problems from which they have previously suffered. I have witnessed many problems relating to circulatory obstruction improve dramatically with chelation therapy, and prefer applying this approach before enlisting some of the invasive therapies currently in use.

3. Hydrotherapy
   A gentle and powerful total-body tonifier that increases the body's immunity, repair and circulatory system. Temperature transfer via the medium of water can decrease the time it normally takes to effect regeneration and restoration. Some hydrotherapeutic benefits are:
   • increasing red blood cell production

- increasing white blood cell production
- increasing overall metabolism
- decreasing total cholesterol
- decreasing triglycerides
- normalizing blood sugar
- decreasing stress hormones
- decreasing blood pressure
- exercising the circulatory system

Many simple techniques can be done in the home shower or tub; others may require a spa or clinic. The concept is simple and the results have been rewarding.

In summary, the treatment of stroke involves a team effort. Orthodoxy is best suited for immediate potentially-life-saving intervention and allaying further progressive damage. Recovery involves a diversified approach, involving the mind, body and spirit. A well-chosen team of health care professionals can provide many beneficial therapies, coupled with genuine support and caring. The patient should be encouraged to become actively involved in the process: to question, participate, and initiate as they are able. The recovery from stroke, as well as from any other illness or disease, is also a matter of the patient's relationship with their spiritual essence, in whatever expression is appropriate for them. This can be learned, enhanced and supported.

Resources:

The American Association of Naturopathic Physicians
P.O. Box 20386
Seattle, WA 98102
(216) 323-7610

World Research Foundation
15300 Ventura Blvd., Suite 405
Sherman Oaks, CA 91403
(818) 907-5483
(Current research information available)

Contributors

Dr. Michael M. Saling PhD, MAPs.S. Senior Lecturer and Convenor of Clinical Neuropsychology—University of Melbourne. Honorary Head, Department of Neuropsychology, Austin Hospital. Was involved in a recently published collaborative study on Striatocapsular Stroke at the Austin Hospital. Has published books on Luria's Aphasiology and Freud's Neurological Writings, and is currently involved in research on memory function in temporal lobe epilepsy.

Carol Burton MA, MAPs.S. Senior Psychologist, Hampton Rehabilitation Hospital. Has been working as a clinical neuropsychologist for 15 years in rehabilitation and private practice. Previously practiced as a vocational and counselling psychologist specializing in rehabilitation. Foundation member, and current member of the National Executive Committee of the Board of Clinical Neuropsychologists of the Australian Psychological Society. Currently undertaking research into the psychological management of pain after burns.

Dr. Geoffrey A. Donnan MD, FRACP. Neurologist at the Austin Hospital, Senior Associate at University of Melbourne, Stroke Unit Austin Hospital. Major interest in cerebrovascular disease.

Dr. Stephen Davis MD, FRACP. Consultant Neurologist and co-ordinator of the Royal Melbourne Hospital Stroke Service. Has a particular interest in stroke research, particularly in the measurement and analysis of cerebral blood flow after particular types of stroke. Also supervises the rehabilitation of stroke patients at the Essendon Rehabilitation Unit of the Amalgamated Melbourne and Essendon Hospitals.

Dr. Graeme Penington MBBS, DPRM, FRACGP, FRACMA, FACRM. Worked as a general practitioner for fourteen years before entering the speciality of Rehabilitation Medicine some thirteen years ago. Director of Rehabilitation, Mount Royal Hospital, Dr. Penington's unit has a major interest in rehabilitation for stroke, disorders of swallowing and amputations. Principal author of a new book— "Introduction to Medical Rehabilitation: an Australasian Perspective".

Heather Mudie DIP.O.T.(NSW), DIP Neuro Sc. Chief Occupational Therapist at Cedar Court Physical Rehabilitation Hospital in Melbourne. Has undertaken extensive studies and research in the Occupational Therapy field. Received AAOT Research Award and was the recipient of the Gwendoline Sims Memorial Award by the NSW Association of Occupational Therapists in 1989.

Mrs. Clare Gray Coordinator of the Australian Brain Foundation's Stroke Assistance Services, including the Stroke Support Scheme. Experience came from 14 years of caring for her mother who suffered a stroke at the age of 50. Has been involved in the establishment of many Stroke Support Groups in Victoria.

Marilyn Collins RN, CNS, CERT IT, DIB Ed Stud (Mon). Extensive experience in health promotion and education, and health service provision with particular expertise in cardiovascular health. Originally trained in nursing with further studies in psychology, education, health and human relations and sociological/organizational theory. Curently Health Service Coordinator of a Community Health Center in Melbourne.

Elizabeth Beringer An authorized Feldenkrais® teacher who has worked in the field of movement education for over fifteen years. She lives and works in Berkeley, California and in addition she travels extensively teaching workshops and in training programs worldwide. She often sees people with orthopedic and neurological problems as well as specializing in working with atheletes. She is the editor of the Feldenkrais Journal.

Marcus Laux N.D., D.Hom (Med). A licensed, practicing naturopathic physician and a graduate of National College of Naturopathic Medicine in Portland, Oregon. Dr. Laux is a nutritional and herbal product formulator, medical consultant, and spokesperson for several health and fitness companies. He has served as an assistant adjunct professor at Emperors College of Traditional Oriental Medicine in Santa Monica, California, and lectures internationally about nutritional and attitudinal health, self-care, and self-responsibility. In private family practice in the Los Angeles area, he uses natural therapeutics and supports his patients by helping them help themselves.

Glossary

agraphia Inability to express thoughts in writing due to a lesion of a particular part of the brain.

alexia Loss of the ability to understand the written word due to a lesion of the brain.

amaurosis fugax Brief blindness in one eye due to a temporary blood vessel lesion.

aneurysm Localised swelling in the wall of the blood vessel.

angiography X-ray test of a blood vessel by the use of radio opaque dye. Used as a diagnostic aid for stroke and other vascular diseases.

aphasia Loss of the ability to speak due to an injury to the brain.

apraxia Loss of the ability to carry out familiar movements in the absence of paralysis.

arteriovenous malformations A clump of distorted blood vessels caused by abnormal connections between arteries and veins.

ataxia Loss of co-ordination and balance.

atherosclerosis A deposit of cholesterol and fatty plaques on the inside of arteries. A very common cause of blocked arteries.

atrial fibrillation Irregular heart rate due to an abnormality of muscular contraction.

biofeedback The ability for a person to modify their own bodily functions eg. blood pressure, pulse by mental relaxation and other techniques.

brain stem Lowest part of the brain connecting the cerebral hemispheres with the spinal cord.

capsulitis Inflamation of the ligaments surrounding a joint; a common complication in a limb paralysed by a stroke.

carotid arteries The pair of main arteries running on each side of the neck supplying blood to the brain.

carotid circulation system The arterial system of blood supply to the front two-thirds of the brain.

CAT scan Computerised Axial Tomography — A common form of X-ray imaging of the brain. Useful in investigation of stroke.

cerebral infarction Damage to brain tissue due to a blocked artery supplying that part of the brain.

cerebral haemorrhage A bleed into the brain due to rupture of a vessel supplying it.

cerebral venous thrombosis A clot blocking a vein draining blood from the brain.

cerebellum Back part of the brain concerned with the co-ordination of movement and balance.

cerebrum The major portion of the brain occupying the upper part of the skull.

deep heat therapy A form of physiotherapy used to relax muscles which have stiffened as an aftermath of paralysis of that limb such as from a stroke.

Doppler ultrasound A method of measuring blood flow through arteries and veins using sound waves.

double vision Seeing two images.

duplex ultrasound A special form of Doppler ultrasound.

dyspraxia Partial loss of the ability to perform familiar movements in the absence of paralysis. (Compare apraxia)

dystrophy A painful degeneration of skin and muscle tissue as an uncommon complication of limb paralysis.

echocardiograph Method of measuring the function and thickness of the heart muscle by use of sound waves.

electrocardiograph Common method of measuring the electrical activity of the heart muscle usually recorded on a graph.

endarterectomy The removal of clot or atheromatus plaque from the inside of an artery.

functional stimulation Electrical stimulation of a nerve or muscle.

hemiparesis Weakness or partial paralysis involving one side of the body.

homonymous heminiopia Loss of vision effecting either right or left halves of the combined visual field of both eyes.

hypertension Raised blood pressure above normal values.

infarction Death of tissue due to a blocked artery supplying it i.e. heart muscle or brain tissue.

lacune A small, usually crescent-shaped, region of infarction deep within the brain substance.

neglect A term used to describe patients who seem unaware of part of their bodies often after a stroke.

occlusion Blockage of a blood vessel.

orthosis A medical appliance used to support deformities of a limb, e.g. a splint.

spasticity Increased tone in muscle groups resulting in stiffened joint movements.

stenosis Narrowing of an artery with consequent reduced blood flow.

stereotactic surgery Precise brain surgery made possible by the use of X-ray imaging.

subarachnoid haemorrhage A particular form of brain haemorrhage occuring between layers covering the brain.

subarachnoid space A space lying between connective tissue membranes covering the brain.

subluxation Incomplete or partial dislocation of a joint.

transient ischaemic attack A temporary insufficiency of blood supply to any region of the brain.

transient monocular blindness Temporary loss of vision in one eye, usually due to a blocked artery.

vertebral arteries Two arteries running up the spine at the back of the neck supplying the back one-third of the brain.

vertebrobasilar circulation system Part of the complex blood supply to the brain — joins up with vessels branching from the carotid arteries.

vertigo Dizziness resulting in loss of balance.

Index